"Excellence"

"Dr. Burdenko has brought water and land therapy to a new level of excellence. Using the methods in his book, individuals with physical disabilities, myself included, no longer have to be handicapped by their disabilities. This book gives those of us who are physically challenged techniques to use to live vital, productive, and active lives."

Diane Roberts Stoler, Ed.D.
author of *Coping With Mild Traumatic Brain Injury*

"Progressive"

"As a rehabilitation therapist for twenty-eight years, I have used many different techniques on my patients to enhance their recovery. The Burdenko Method presented in *Overcoming Paralysis* is progressive, sequential, and provides results beyond one's expectations. The outcome is the ability to live life more fully, whether in a wheelchair or competing in an Olympic event."

Paula G. Ray
President, Rehab Focus, Inc.

"Never Give Up Hope"

"In 1995 at the age of 45, I was hit by a car while riding my bicycle. My doctors and physical therapists had given up all hope on my chances of being able to walk unassisted again. Then I met Igor Burdenko and followed his program. With his help, I am able to walk, swim, run, and bike again. If you have ever suffered a serious injury, this book may teach you to never give up hope. I lay paralyzed and wondered if I would ever walk again. The program laid out in this book helped me to get my life back. Use it to regain yours."

Andrew Geller
M.D., M.P.H

OVERCOMING
PARALYSIS

IGOR BURDENKO, PhD
SCOTT BIEHLER

AVERY PUBLISHING GROUP

Garden City Park • New York

The therapeutic procedures in this book are based on the training, personal experiences, and research of the authors. Because each person and situation is unique, the author and publisher urge the reader to check with a qualified health professional before using any procedure where there is any question to its appropriateness.

The publisher does not advocate the use of any particular treatment, but believes the information presented in this book should be available to the public.

Because there is always some risk involved, the author and publisher are not responsible for any adverse effects or consequences resulting from the use of any of the suggestions or procedures described in this book. This book is as timely and accurate as its publisher and authors can make it; nevertheless, they disclaim all liability and cannot be held responsible for any problems that may arise from its use. Please do not use the book if you are unwilling to assume the risk. Feel free to consult with a physician or other qualified health professional. It is a sign of wisdom, not cowardice, to seek a second or third opinion.

Cover designer: Phaedra Mastrocola
In-house editor: Dara Stewart
Typesetter: Gary A. Rosenberg
Illustrator: Scott Biehler
Printer: Paragon Press, Honesdale, PA

Avery Publishing Group
120 Old Broadway
Garden City Park, NY 11040
1–800–548–5757
www.averypublishing.com

Wet Vest is a registered trademark of Bioenergetics.
Hydro-Fit is a registered trademark of Hydro-Fit Incorporated.
The Water Workout Station is a registered trademark of the Aquatrend Company.

Library of Congress Cataloging-in-Publication Data

Burdenko, Igor.
  Overcoming paralysis: into the water and out of the wheelchair / Igor Burdenko, Scott Biehler.
    p. cm.
  Includes bibliographical references and index.
  ISBN 0-89529-883-X
    1. Paralytics—Rehabilitation.   2. Paraplegia—Exercise therapy.   3. Quadriplegia—Exercise therapy.   4. Aquatic exercises.
    I. Biehler, Scott.   II. Title.
  RC406.P3B87   1999
  362.4'38-dc21   99-20886
                                                                        CIP

Printed in the United States of America

10   9   8   7   6   5   4   3   2   1

Contents

PART THREE   Water Exercises

Acknowledgments

We are grateful to the following individuals and companies who helped make this book possible through their support: Mr. and Mrs. David B. Arnold, Jr.; Helen H. Ayer; Steve and Joan Belkin; DeVasto Associates; Jan Durgin; Priscilla Endicott; Myrna and Gene Freedman; Dr. Andrew Geller; Finn and Joyce Hals; Philip C. Haughey; Larry and Sarah Holden; Dr. and Mrs. Stephen H. Kapin; Martin and Wendy Kaplan; Mun Ryoung Kim; Joan Klagsbrun; Barbara and Tom Leggat; Deborah Smith Leighton; Ken and Abby MacPherson; Paul Maki; Tracy and Kathy Mallory; Glenn McWaters of Bioenergetics, Inc.; Julian Miller; Mr. and Mrs. Stanley Miller; Kristina O'Conor; Leon Okurowski; Susan Palmateer; Harold and Edith Rosenberg; Richard and Mary Rosenblatt; Diane Rothhammer of Sprint Rothhammer International; Dr. Michael A. Rubin; William B. Russell; Karen and Steven Salhaney; Jeff Schoenherr of J and B Foam Fabricators, Inc.; Chuck Schwager; Richard Suarez; Mr. and Mrs. Thurow; Dr. and Mrs. Joseph Upton; and Paul S. Wylie.

We would also like to thank Steven Blauer for his help, support, and belief in us; and Dara Stewart for her outstanding skills in communication and her professionalism.

Preface

It has been estimated that there are 150,000 wheelchair users as the result of spinal-cord injury in the United States today. It is hoped that in the next ten years, researchers will find a medical breakthrough that will lead to an ultimate cure. The plight of Christopher Reeve (the actor who portrayed Superman in the movies) has brought much attention to the efforts of researchers trying to find a cure for paralysis. For those who have to deal with paralysis now, the medical profession has little to offer in the way of recovery.

While scientists have been spending millions of dollars on research, one man has quietly been achieving results rehabilitating the paralyzed through his innovative techniques. I was lucky enough to find out about his accomplishments and to have the opportunity to work with him.

Dr. Igor Burdenko has incorporated his years of study and practical results into a program of rehabilitation and conditioning called the Burdenko Method. It is a comprehensive approach of working with the whole body, not just the injury, with a special emphasis on stimulating and exercising the body in the water as well as on the land.

This book is written as a practical application of the Burdenko Method to help wheelchair users who have been paralyzed overcome the difficulties they experience and improve the quality of their everyday lives. It provides a realistic approach to dealing with the physical and mental problems wheelchair users encounter with their health due to being confined to a wheelchair. The book encompasses Dr. Burdenko's positive philosophy of helping the body heal itself and of the benefits of using a combination of water and land exercises. It explores the special qualities of water when used as a modality for rehabilitation and conditioning.

SCOTT BIEHLER'S STORY

At the age of 41, I was enjoying a career as an account manager for a computer graphics company in the Boston area. My wife, my two sons, aged 9 and 16, and I had just finished an active summer. We had been blue-fishing on Martha's Vineyard and hiking in the Grand Tetons; we had visited Yellowstone and attended a National Wildlife Federation family summit in Big Sky, Montana.

I've had a passion for riding motorcycles since I was a young boy. Over the years I have owned a variety of different models and was thrilled to have just gotten a Ninja ZX-10. I had owned the motorcycle for about two months when I took it for a ride on a lovely autumn afternoon. I was trying to impress one of my friends, and while going around a curve, I lost control. The next thing I remember, I was on my way to the hospital in a helicopter. I had broken my back and was paralyzed from the chest down.

Since my accident, all the medical evaluations have been the same. I was told that, short of a medical breakthrough, I will not be able to walk again. I have been told that in order to get on with my life, I need to be able to accept my fate and learn to live with my limitations.

To add to my "misfortune," I have chronic pain that seems to be incurable as well. After visiting several neurosurgeons, I was finally told that my life was going to be different now. I would have to accept the fact that I could only look forward to accomplishing a small percentage of my goals. I'd have to learn to settle for less, since that is all I would be capable of achieving. Essentially, I have been told that I am a subset of my former self.

Boy, talk about bedside manner! Some doctors were cruelly blunt, painting a bleak picture of the future. Others were polite, and tried to candy-coat their words, but the message was still the same. No wonder people stay paralyzed. Just listen to the messages we get.

I kept hoping that I'd find a doctor who was smarter than the rest or knew something the others didn't. I pursued the normal channels for rehabilitation, including an endless stream of medical specialists, therapists, medications, traditional treatments, and alternative methods of healing. My family and I moved from the Boston suburbs to northern New Hampshire, in hopes that the fresh air and peaceful setting would help me rest and give my body time to heal. The people who sold us our home asked if we had moved here to work with Dr. Burdenko. They assumed that I knew of his accomplishments in working with handicapped people and that I had come to visit his institute in Waterville Valley, New Hampshire, The Burdenko Water and Sports Therapy Institute. This was how I first learned of Dr. Burdenko. He and I subsequently met to discuss my situation, and I discovered that he has helped other people in my situation recover from paralysis. So I stumbled upon this doctor quite by chance.

Dr. Burdenko has a whole philosophy on the way in which the human body heals from injury. He has developed a method of rehabilitation over the years that encompasses taking care of the whole body, with an emphasis on the use of water therapy. He treats his patients as though they were athletes in training, trying to get their bodies into the best possible condition. He believes and has proven that the body has the power to heal itself. This can be achieved by conditioning the mind with the proper attitude and taking care of your body with nutrition and the appropriate exercise.

When Dr. Burdenko and I began working together, I couldn't even maintain my balance to sit up straight. My muscles were weak, and I had difficulty getting around and transferring to and from the wheelchair. I discovered that working out in the water was fun. I was able to move my body with less pain and with greater flexibility in the water. Within months, my strength and stability had dramatically improved. After six months, my wife saw my legs begin to move in the water for the first time. We laughed, and we cried. It was a small movement, but it was something the doctors said would never happen.

I have been elated with my progress so far. I have regained control of some of the muscles below my injury and am looking forward to making further recovery. The best thing for me, as a result of working with Dr. Burdenko, has been the change in my motivation and attitude. His program has paid off many times over in my personal satisfaction alone.

DR. BURDENKO'S STORY

Educated in Russia, Dr. Burdenko received his M.S. in Physical Education and Ph.D. in Sports Medicine. He was working as a professional coach in 1973 when he had an experience that changed the direction of his career. One of his friends was a very talented athlete, training for competition in gymnastics. While high in the air, practicing his elements on the balance beam, his safety belt broke. He land-ed on the beam, breaking his back. The once-strong athlete was left quadriplegic. The only action he could perform was to use a pencil with his mouth. From that point on, Dr. Burdenko has taken a special interest in helping the handicapped. Finding no books and little information on the subject, Igor began adapting his program to address the special needs of the physically challenged. Before leaving Russia, he was able to help his friend regain the use of his arms and write with his hands again.

Dr. Burdenko's first experience working with the handicapped for the special Olympics began in 1983. He based his rehabilitation method on the techniques he learned in Russia, which he used on athletes recovering from sports injuries. He began designing a pro-gram for wheelchair users, which led to his participation as a coach and rehabilitation specialist for athletes in the 1984 World Handicapped Games in Stoke Mandville, England. This experience created a new awareness for helping others.

Dr. Burdenko says: "I have built upon my experience and devel-oped a method that I have found to be effective in helping people recover from their injuries. It is a thrill for me to see my patients improve their physical condition, recover from their injuries, and in many cases, even regain the use of their paralyzed bodies. Working with the handicapped always provides a source of great joy and per-sonal satisfaction."

WHY DID WE WRITE THIS BOOK?

After hearing "No" so many times from doctors and specialists, it is refreshing and exciting to find a program that really helps. I (Scott) knew that there would be thousands of people just like me who have been looking for what I found. So I set out to spread the word. I called several organizations and professional magazines to tell them my exciting news. I was surprised at their lukewarm reception. They were skeptical about a natural method of healing and were reluctant to pursue it with an article. One editor even told me that his maga-zine did not want to get its readers' hopes up about nontraditional treatments. So the next logical step was to document our experience and make it directly available to others who find themselves in a sim-ilar situation. This book has provided an opportunity to share Dr. Burdenko's methods and techniques, which have worked for me.

Dr. Burdenko has achieved extraordinary results at his institute helping people recover from injury and paralysis. He is not the type of person who seeks fame or recognition, but he has a desire to share his knowledge. He would like to make his methods available to as many people as possible. His work has been featured in Boston newspapers and on local television, but it still remains unknown to most wheelchair users for whom it could provide the most benefit.

This book is an opportunity to share our success with as many wheelchair users as possible and provide them with hope and inspiration to improve their health and, we hope, even recover from their injuries.

DR. BURDENKO'S PHILOSOPHY

I am 64 years old, and have spent almost four decades working in the fields of rehabilitation, conditioning, and training. I have learned a wide variety of techniques in different countries and at many institutions. I have searched for the best and most efficient techniques to help my patients, students, and clients. After years of experience comparing all the different modalities, I have concluded that working with the whole body (not just the injury), using a combination of water and land exercises without pain, consistently produces the best results in a very safe and enjoyable way.

I religiously believe that people who are handicapped or injured can generate the natural healing process in their bodies through exercise more than with anything else. I have found this to be more effective than pills, surgery, or traditional modalities. When you exercise, you change your body's chemistry. This helps create the best environment to generate the healing process.

The use of water therapy has always been an important part of my life's work in rehabilitation, conditioning, and training. When asked if I could achieve the same results without using the water, I reply that my experience has been that the progress would be much, much slower, and it would be more difficult to achieve the same level of recovery.

An essential part of recovering and staying well is maintaining the right attitude. For this, I have a simple philosophy—The five Fs:

1. Future—Life without a future is senseless.

2. Fitness—If we are not fit and able to function, we cannot enjoy living.

3. Fun—We need to enjoy ourselves! For me, this is the biggest F, because life without fun is somber and dull.

4. Family and Friends—We need to share the excitement of our lives with the people important to us.

5. Fantastic!—When you have the first four Fs, then you are automatically fantastic !

HOW THIS BOOK IS ORGANIZED

This book is written from my (Scott's) point of view, so wheelchair users can directly identify with my situation. The book is divided into three main parts. Part One provides information about recovering from injury with the proper rehabilitation and conditioning. We begin with an explanation of the Burdenko Method and how it is used to help generate the natural healing process, and why this is so effective in restoring nerve damage. Then, we discuss the importance of using water as a therapeutic modality and the characteristics of this wonderful medium that make it ideal for rehabilitation. Next, we cover the basic conditioning principles and techniques that were an essential part of my program and have become a part of my new lifestyle. Special consideration is given to common problems that accompany paralysis, including dealing with pain and depression.

Part Two describes the wheelchair exercises used on the land. Part Three is dedicated to exercising in the water. There are well over 100 exercises with detailed drawings and step-by-step instructions. We emphasize the techniques that Dr. Burdenko taught me to wake up the nerves and muscles in the lower body and eventually to walk in the water. The comments that accompany the exercises are useful for the wheelchair user and for the physical therapists and healthcare professionals who are their coaches and helpers.

Dr. Burdenko has helped many handicapped people recover from their injuries—people like Paul Carney and Bob McKenna, who were quadriplegic and now walk. Their stories are inspiring, and are included along with other testimonies throughout the book.

Introduction

If you are paralyzed and have been seeking a way to improve your physical condition and to aid recovery from your injuries, this book is for you. It is ideally suited for paraplegics or quadriplegics with limited arm use. The same techniques for rehabilitation and conditioning described in this book can be of great value to wheelchair users with other conditions as well.

There are many reasons that people must use wheelchairs, including injury (including spinal-cord damage and limb amputation), illness (polio; multiple sclerosis; Guillain-Barré syndrome) and declining health due to physical inactivity. Movement into, out of, and inside the wheelchair is largely controlled by the arms and upper-body muscles. You may find your ability to move around independently is limited by a lack of strength and endurance. Additionally, wheelchair users often suffer from a sedentary lifestyle causing limited range of motion, stiff joints, and muscle degradation (atrophy). People with all of these problems can benefit by using the reconditioning experience and exercises explained in this book.

If you desire to change your life, and you are not afraid to try new directions, this book will help. It has been our experience that the techniques Dr. Burdenko has perfected can be used to help the body heal itself. He has worked with quadriplegics and paraplegics who have been told that they will never walk again. By applying his method of rehabilitation, some have been able to walk and no longer require the use of their wheelchairs. It takes determination and hard work, but we believe it can be accomplished! So it makes sense to try.

Although an essential part of this program involves rehabilitation

1

in the water, this book is not aimed at people who are swimmers. In fact, you do not have to know how to swim at all. The activities in the water are all done with floatation devices. Water is used as a modality to aid in rehabilitation, conditioning, and recovery.

It is well accepted that all people can benefit from a program of physical and strength conditioning. Recent studies have shown that people who exercise vigorously tend to live longer and have better health. There are no exceptions to this, regardless of age or physical limitations. Taking care of one's body is just as important for wheelchair users as it is for anyone else. Our main purpose is to educate the body to function safely, gracefully, and efficiently.

The Burdenko Method for recovery following an injury and for physical conditioning is threefold. First, we need to take care of our health with proper breathing, eating, and liquid intake. Second, we must work on the abilities we need for everyday life. We rebuild balance, coordination, flexibility, endurance, strength, and speed. Third, we must help the body heal itself by stimulating and attempting to wake up the damaged muscles and nerves. Most programs of exercise refer to the old phrase: "Use it or lose it." This takes on special meaning for physically challenged individuals who may have already "lost it" as a result of an injury.

Recovery from one's injuries and the motivation to heal are directly related. Using the Burdenko Method, physically handicapped people have been able to regain the use of their bodies, even after a medical diagnosis indicated otherwise. People who have been told that there is no possibility of a full recovery have beaten the odds and been able to significantly improve their health and mobility. The desire to be independent is a powerful driving mechanism for the physically challenged. Time and again, people who follow the Burdenko Method have improved their health and have had tremendous results recovering from their injuries.

Our main purpose is to educate the body to function safely, gracefully, and efficiently. Special consideration is given to working with the whole body, not just the injury. This book is about changing your thinking to help the body heal itself and to develop an ongoing maintenance plan for a healthy lifestyle. This includes the power of positive thinking, the power of exercising, the power of diet therapy, and the power of pain management. These are the important aspects of conditioning the handicapped.

We cannot guarantee that the Burdenko Method outlined in this book will solve all your problems or that you will fully recover. What we can say is that for many people, the Burdenko Method has worked where all other options have failed. We hope it will work for you. The degree to which you can succeed will vary. The important thing is that you never give up! You can achieve results. With the right attitude, we feel there are no limits on what you may be able to achieve using the Burdenko Method. We believe that only the body can heal itself. Our goal is to provide an environment in which the body can do its work.

Our main concern is your safety. You should consult your physician or physical therapist before following any of the recommendations in this book. A health-care professional who understands your condition and knows your fitness level should ensure that this material is appropriate for you.

Adapting the techniques that he has used to help professional athletes recover from sport injuries, Dr. Burdenko has developed a unique method of land and water therapy for handicapped people. This book documents his new and creative methods, specifically adapted for wheelchair users. It provides the hope, inspiration, and mental and physical conditioning techniques needed for those seeking to improve their health.

The first chapter explains what goes wrong that causes paralysis. It includes a discussion of the physiology of the spine and the nervous system.

A full chapter is dedicated to explaining the Burdenko Method. This is Dr. Burdenko's program for conditioning and rehabilitation that he first pioneered in Russia and later developed in the United States over the past thirty-five years.

The importance of using water therapy in rehabilitation is addressed next. The benefits of exercising in the water are explored, with a review of the physical properties that make water an ideal medium for conditioning.

Next, we get into the meat of the book and start discussing how to take care of your health through proper eating and conditioning principles. This provides the foundation for the exercises that will follow. Special consideration is given to problems that are common following a severe injury, including dealing with pain and depression.

Designing a personal rehabilitation plan is the next step. A detailed description of my particular program provides a reference for customizing your own plan.

The latter portion of the book is dedicated to the actual exercises. These are divided into land (wheelchair) and water exercises. The exercises are generally ordered from simple to complex.

At the end of the book, you will find a detailed bibliography, which provides a source of materials for supplementary reading and future reference, and a list of the equipment described in the book with the manufacturers' names and addresses.

Some people naturally have an amazing will to overcome their circumstances. I remember watching the movie about Dennis Byrd, the football player who was paralyzed in a head-on collision during a game. When he was told he would never walk again, he made up his mind that he was not going to accept that diagnosis. He decided that he would walk again, in spite of the medical predictions. He was determined to get better, and miraculously, he overcame his paralysis and recovered. He had what most of us have had stripped away— hope and a belief that we will get better.

When the medical prognosis says, "No," Dr. Burdenko says, "Yes." *Overcoming Paralysis* offers hope to the wheelchair community. This book is the food for those who hunger for information on how to get better. This is a practical application with proven techniques that work. Physical therapists and health practitioners who are involved in rehabilitation and conditioning will also find this book to be a valuable reference manual. It will help in motivating and structuring a rehabilitation program for physically challenged people according to their present condition and realistic goals.

Don't believe it when someone tells you that there is nothing else that can be done to improve your situation. Limitations on your thinking are what make you handicapped. Negative thinking puts limits on your ability and progress. If you have limitations—do not accept them. No one knows the boundaries of the human potential. You can exceed your current limitations and progress to achieve goals that you set in your mind.

Life is movement. Never stop moving. Don't lie in bed saying, "I tried it, and it didn't work." Keep an open mind and try many different directions. Keep trying over and over again. Never give up! Work hard with a smile. Exercise as much as you can for your mind and body.

Each person has his or her own unique problems following an injury. Initially, the body needs time to rest and recover from the shock and trauma of the accident. The recovery for each person will vary based on his or her physical and mental state. Some people need time to deal with their new situation while others are eager to get started on their rehabilitation.

It would be wonderful to proclaim that the Burdenko Method will cure all injuries, but that would be unrealistic. Why some people are able to overcome insurmountable damage and have their bodies heal themselves and why other people do not is still a mystery to doctors. We do know that a positive mental attitude and conditioning play essential roles in the healing process and recovery. This is something I have experienced myself.

There are different degrees of recovery. Any improvement in pain relief, attitude, balance, coordination, flexibility, endurance, strength, or speed is a step toward recovery. We always seem to want what we don't have. The trick is to set realistic goals and participate in a program of activity to achieve them. You can revise your goals from time to time based on the full understanding of what you have been able to achieve along the way.

The Burdenko Method encourages you first to accomplish simple tasks. As your body improves, you will see the results and set more strenuous goals. This book can be used as a guide for people whose ultimate goal is regaining full use of their bodies. The extent of your recovery depends on your determination and ability.

PART ONE

The Background of the Burdenko Method

ONE

Understanding Paralysis

Simply speaking, paralysis is the loss of muscle use and/or sensation. The primary cause of paralysis is a spinal-cord injury, commonly referred to as an SCI. Spinal-cord injuries are often caused by vehicular accidents, severe falls, and gunshot injuries. Less commonly, paralysis may be caused by such conditions as infection, compression of the spinal cord, spina bifida, stroke, or cysts or tumors growing on the spine. In order to understand paralysis and its causes, let's first take a look at the spine and the nervous system.

THE SPINE

The spine is a complex part of the body, comprised of the backbone and spinal cord. The spinal cord is the means by which the brain broadcasts messages to the rest of the body and vice versa. It is a group of nerves extending downward from the brain, with nerves branching out along the entire cord. The spinal cord is protected by the bones of the spinal column, or backbone. The individual bones of the spinal column are called vertebrae.

The spinal column can be divided into four areas: the cervical, thoracic, lumbar, and sacral regions, and the coccyx, which is composed of four vertebrae fused together. There are thirty-three vertebrae. The seven vertebrae in the neck compose the cervical region. The twelve vertebrae just below the neck and above the lower back compose the thoracic area. The vertebrae in the lower back compose the lumbar area. The tailbone is comprised of five bones fused together. This is called the sacrum. The vertebrae in each area of the spine are numbered starting from the top. The first cervical vertebra at the base of the skull is numbered C-1, and the last cervical vertebra is numbered C-7. The thoracic vertebrae are numbered T-1 through T-12, the lumbar vertebrae are numbered L-1 through L-5, and the sacral vertebrae are numbered S-1 through S-5.

THE NERVOUS SYSTEM

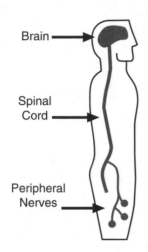

Figure 1.1.
The nervous system.

We control movement in our bodies through signals sent and received through the nervous system. There are two main parts of the nervous system: the central nervous system and the peripheral nervous system. The central nervous system is composed of the brain and the spinal cord. The peripheral nervous system is composed of a network of nerves extending from the spinal cord to the rest of the body. (See Figure 1.1, left.)

Nerve signals travel in two directions. Thoughts originate in our brains and are coded into signals that proceed down the spinal cord and out through the peripheral nerves. These signals then tell our arms to move or our legs to walk or our bodies to do whatever it is that we want them to do. Likewise, our hands or other parts of our bodies touch something hot or feel pressure or taste something sweet, and then send a signal to the brain, which interprets that signal as heat, pressure, or sweetness. All of this happens in a fraction of a second via the nervous system.

The cells of the nervous system are called neurons. (See Figure 1.2 on page 11.) Each of these nerve cells has a large body with a long extension called an axon, which sends messages, and several extensions called dendrites, which receive messages. The space between the axon of one neuron and the dendrite of another is called a synapse. It is across this space that neurons transmit messages.

Neurons send messages by means of electrical currents with the help of some chemicals. At the synapse, the axon secretes chemicals called neurotransmitters, which convey the electrical current containing its message. (See Figure 1.3 on page 11.) The current is then passed on to the dendrite of the next neuron, so that this cell can receive and pass on the message. Different nerves use different types of neurotransmitters to transmit different messages.

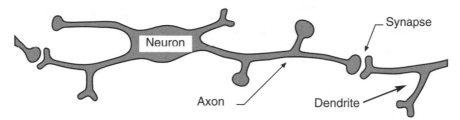

Figure 1.2. A neuron.

PARALYSIS

When there is injury to the spinal column, the nerves of the spinal cord are damaged or severed, interrupting the flow of messages being communicated between the brain and the rest of the body. When the brain cannot communicate with the body's members, paralysis is the result.

Spinal-cord injuries are usually classified as complete or incomplete. These classifications refer to the severity of the injury. With complete spinal-cord injury, the nerves passing through the affected area are completely damaged. Doctors usually tell the patient that there is little to no hope for recovery of use and sensation with complete spinal-cord injury.

Injury to different parts of the spinal cord cause different types of paralysis. Injury to the area between C-1 and C-5 is the most devastating. It causes paralysis of the arm and leg muscles, as well as the muscles needed for breathing. It is usually fatal. Injury to the C-5 to C-7 vertebrae causes paralysis of the legs and some paralysis of the arms. Injury to any of the thoracic vertebrae causes paralysis of the legs and varying degrees of paralysis of the trunk. Injury of the lumbar and the S-1 to S-2 vertebrae causes some type of leg weakness and numbness, and injury to the S-3 to S-5 vertebrae causes loss of bladder and bowel control, and loss of feeling in the anal region.

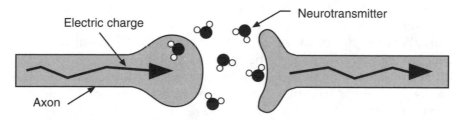

Figure 1.3. Communication between neurons.

Paralysis is generally categorized as one of three types—paraplegia, quadriplegia, and hemiplegia.

Paraplegia

Paraplegia is paralysis of the lower portion of the body, particularly the legs. The back and the abdominal muscles may be affected as well. Symptoms include loss of motion, sensation, and reflexes below the level of damage immediately following injury. With complete spinal-cord injury, a patient may lose bladder and bowel control and sexual function.

Quadriplegia

Quadriplegia is paralysis of the body below the level of injury, as well as of the arms and legs. Quadriplegia is usually the result of an injury to the spinal cord in the area between the fifth and the seventh vertebrae.

Hemiplegia

Hemiplegia is paralysis affecting one side of the body. Infantile hemiplegia affects infants as a result of insufficient oxygen received in the womb, a brain hemorrhage at birth, or a fever during infancy. Cerebral hemiplegia is the result of a brain tumor.

HOW THE NERVOUS SYSTEM HEALS

Nerve cells require a constant supply of blood, which provides the oxygen and nutrients that allow the cells to function properly. Without oxygen, the neurons degrade, and if the oxygen is cut off for too long, eventually the cells will die. In the case of spinal-cord injury, nerves are usually not severed, but instead suffer damage from bruising and swelling that restricts adequate blood supply.

When the blood supply is replenished, the neurons attempt to repair themselves. In living neurons, the axons return to their healthy state, allowing communication to be restored. If the neurons have been permanently damaged, the nervous system tries to bypass the old network to establish alternate communication links. As the healthy nerves are stimulated, new axons branch out and send out neurotransmitters. (See Figure 1.4 on page 13.) The dendrites of other neurons are attracted to these neurotransmitters, causing the neurons to link up.

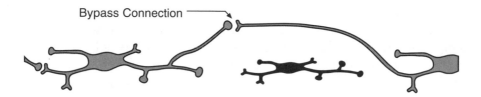

Bypass Connection

Figure 1.4. The nervous system's establishment of alternate communication links.

The ability of the neurons to branch out appears to be influenced by the amount of stimulation they receive. With a constant supply of electrical impulses, the axons strive to reconnect. When the stimulus slows down or disappears, the nerve activity ceases. This combination of electrical and chemical transmission provides the instructions to enhance natural healing.

Nerves can be stimulated physically by exercise. The thought to move originates in the brain and gets sent as a signal down the nervous system and out to the muscles. During massage, or when an assistant is helping you exercise, the sensation of the touching and movement of your body is picked up by the peripheral nerves, and the signal is sent back to the brain. So the exercise is stimulating the nerves by sending and receiving signals. Mental stimulation also causes your body to produce certain chemicals to transmit signals. Feelings of joy, sadness, and fear may cause your body to produce such chemicals as endorphins, the body's natural painkillers. Other chemicals produced in response to mental stimulation send signals to release nerve growth factors.

So the way to enhance the healing process is to provide stimulation, both physically and mentally.

The use of steroids has been effective in many cases in preventing paralysis if administered within twenty-four hours of an SCI. Steroids help reduce swelling and promote healing of the neurons, but their efficacy differs from patient to patient and depends upon the extent of the injury.

Some people who suffer an SCI are able to recover shortly after their accident. If the swelling is controlled and the neurons in the spinal cord do not die, function will most likely return as the neurons heal. In some cases, healthy neurons will branch out and extend themselves to bypass damaged cells and reconnect to other healthy neurons.

Much of today's medical research for a cure for paralysis caused by a spinal-cord injury looks at ways to stimulate the growth of nerve cells or surgically replace damaged nerve cells with new ones. As explained later in this book, Dr. Burdenko believes that many people who suffered an SCI have the power to heal themselves by stimulating nerve growth and regeneration through use of the Burdenko Method.

TWO

The Burdenko Method

D r. Burdenko has achieved great success in helping people recover from injury. After thirty-five years of experience in sports medicine, physical therapy, rehabilitation, and physical conditioning, he has incorporated his studies into a program called the Burdenko Method. The Burdenko Method is not a random set of exercises. It is a system with a history, a philosophy, and levels of development. In this chapter, we will explore how the program was developed and its key points.

THE BACKGROUND OF THE BURDENKO METHOD

As a young boy growing up in Russia, Igor Burdenko was very interested in sports. He played hard, and, like most young athletes, he occasionally had some injuries. During World War II, Igor's father had been wounded five times. The only reason he survived was that he had exercised all his life, was very athletic, and had been in great shape. Igor saw his father swimming and doing exercises in the water frequently and wondered how he could function in the water with all his injuries. When asked how this was possible, his father replied that it was the only way he could get relief from his pain. This fascinated Igor. He started exercising in the water, doing the routine his father had shown him. He discovered that exercising in the water was fun. He also learned that after an injury he could exercise in the water with much less pain and that the recovery time was significantly less. This sparked an interest that led to using the water as a therapeutic means throughout Igor's career.

Igor's fascination in health and fitness continued, and as a young man he competed in state and national cross-country and speed-skating events. After obtaining his degrees in Physical Education and Sports Medicine, Dr. Burdenko worked professionally as a coach. He became interested in establishing a scientific study to test the techniques he had developed, using water therapy to condition and rehabilitate his athletes. Dr. Burdenko headed a research project sponsored by the government department of Ministry of Sports and Education. Members of the project included engineers, medical doctors, orthopedic specialists, athletes, biochemists, physicists, a dermatologist, an obstetrician, and many other professionals. The goal was to bring to 300 million Russians a program that would help in:

- Conditioning for able-bodied people to maintain good health.

- Training for athletes.

- Rehabilitation from injuries.

The studies began with chickens, cats, pigs, dogs, dolphins, and other animals. It then progressed to people from young children through adults. The tests and experiments were conducted on both the healthy and the injured. Much of their study focused on athletes who, almost by nature, push the limits, are well organized, and are disciplined in their approach to physical fitness. Their research proved that animals and people recover from injury faster and develop their muscles better exercising in the water, compared with a control group who practiced traditionally on land. Parts of this program were then used to condition top Russian athletes.

After twenty years as a specialist in rehabilitation and training in Russia, Dr. Burdenko moved to the United States in 1981 where he has continued to develop his program. His research has included studies of different theories and treatments from the ancient past up through the current practices of today. He has traveled the world to observe and test different modalities and techniques in rehabilitation for maintaining a state of good health. During the last eighteen years in Boston, he has refined his techniques, working to condition professional athletes as well as rehabilitate people recovering from severe injury. The Burdenko Method has evolved into a program of health and exercise that has five key points.

THE FIVE KEY POINTS OF THE BURDENKO METHOD

It takes hard work and dedication to get your body into a state of good health and fitness. The Burdenko Method conditions the whole body in order to bring it into a state of health and fitness. This can be achieved by focusing on the following key points.

Work in the Water and on Land

Water has special qualities that make it ideal for rehabilitation therapy. (This will be discussed in greater detail in Chapter 3.) Exercise in the water is an essential part of the Burdenko Method, as you put less stress on the body while working. When recovering from injury, it is usually best to start rehabilitation in the deep water with a flotation vest or belt, where your body can float without any restrictions. You begin by learning to stretch and relax. Then you will work into a series of exercises as will be described in Parts Two and Three of this book.

As you use water exercises as a gentle means of stimulating and reconditioning the body, you will also be doing a routine on the land. The land-based exercises described in this book are designed to be performed in the wheelchair. Many of the exercises are first performed in the water, where it is more relaxing and easier to move. Once you have mastered the exercises in the water, similar exercises are performed on land. Exercises out of the water are more demanding, as you will experience the full effect of gravity on the body. As you progress in your rehabilitation, the water exercises move to shallower water, where you begin to support some body weight. At the same time, the land-based exercises become more challenging.

Eventually, you will transition to performing most of the exercises on the land. As you regain the use of your body, the cycle reverses and you will begin doing more challenging exercises in the water to build up endurance and strength with the help of the resistance of the water.

Depending on your level of recovery, you will spend more or less time in the water, but you will always use a combination of both water- and land-based exercises. Exercises are usually more effective when performed outdoors. There is more oxygen in the air, it is more pleasant outside, and you feel less tired. So whenever possible, exercise outside in the fresh air, both in the water and on the land.

Work in the Vertical Position in the Water

The vertical position is the natural human functioning position. When you are upright, your spine and internal organs are in their natural positions. In rehabilitation, conditioning, and training, the body works best in the vertical position to achieve its full potential in the water. This is especially important for people with paraplegia and quadriplegia. Wearing a flotation vest or belt in the water, you can maintain the upright vertical position with little or no effort.

Most traditional exercise routines for paraplegics are conducted sitting or lying on an exercise mat or in the wheelchair. This is not the natural position for exercise and physical conditioning. Exercising in the water in the vertical position allows you to retrain the body to return to its natural position while the healing process occurs.

Work With the Whole Body

Physical therapists and doctors tend to focus their attention primarily on the location of the injury. However, it is important to work on the whole body. It is just as important to consider the function of your heart, lungs, and liver—the whole body as one unit—as it is to work on the injury. When you improve the function of the whole body, the healing process can start. In the human body, there are more than 650 muscles. It is the goal of the Burdenko Method to reach and develop all of them, working together in harmony.

Good nutrition plays an equally important part in working with the whole body. The quality of the food you consume and the air you breathe determines what nutrients and compounds your body will have to fuel its self-healing process. Not only is what you eat important, but how you eat is also important. (This will be discussed in more detail in Chapter 4.)

The mind is an important part of the whole body as well. Just as the body needs nutrition and exercise, the mind needs to be educated to meditate, control pain, and deal with stress and other demanding situations. The belief that your body has both the power to generate and the ability to visualize the healing process taking place are essential elements of the Burdenko Method.

It is important to recondition the whole body, particularly in the case of paralysis. Much attention will be paid to moving, massaging, and exercising the paralyzed muscles and stimulating the nerves, but that is only part of the rehabilitation process. Exercises for the paralyzed limbs are important, but so, too, is stimulation of the entire body to permit the healing process to function.

Work in Both Directions

We have more than 200 muscles in our bodies that work together in pairs. We need to balance the exercises to equally develop all the muscles. If they are not equally developed, you will have poor coordination and balance. Developing muscles in both directions builds incredible strength and body harmony. This is especially true for wheelchair users. How often do you see a wheelchair going backwards? Traditional rehab techniques often overlook the importance of balancing the muscle development. Any exercise or movement that occurs in one direction should also be performed in the opposite direction.

After an injury or as we grow old, we may use parts of our bodies less and less. This limits the movements of our joints and our range of motion. We find that we are no longer able to do the things we could do before. This is primarily because we move our joints in one direction. When we work in both directions, it helps to more efficiently increase balance, coordination, flexibility, and range of motion.

Work to Develop Six Essential Abilities for Everyday Life and Sport

The program you will follow to develop fitness and return to a state of excellent health occurs with a logical progression of exercises. You need to build up one quality before you can proceed to the next. The first step is to perform exercises to maintain balance. The next progression is to achieve coordination and flexibility. Then move on to endurance exercises, where you build up stamina. As your physical condition improves, the next progression is to work on improving your speed. And finally, exercise for strength to condition and tone the muscles.

Balance

One of the first abilities we develop as infants is the ability to maintain our balance. Balance plays such an essential role in our daily functioning that we tend to take it for granted. As people grow old, they often lose this quality very quickly. For wheelchair users, especially following an injury, maintaining stability may be difficult. Even if the muscles are strong, you cannot function properly without good balance. You need to be able to hold the body erect and make controlled movements without wobbling or falling. Without balance, you cannot properly develop strength and endurance. No matter how good your balance is, it is important to always concentrate on improving it.

Coordination

Coordination is the ability to work your body parts together harmoniously. To move your body uniformly and perform the activities you desire, your muscles need to work together, properly flexing and extending in coordination. Additionally, your muscles and tendons need to be able to move your bones through the full range of motion that your joints allow. As the human body grows from infancy, it acquires coordination through normal development. Your movement becomes an unconscious activity. When you have lost the ability to move due to an injury, illness, or lack of exercise, you have to relearn how to control your movement. Due to lack of motion, your movements become stiff and uncoordinated. You cannot move the way you used to because the muscles are not getting the right signals, and the joints are not flexible. Reconditioning becomes a conscious activity where you focus on each muscle and joint.

For wheelchair users who have limited use of their legs or other parts of their bodies, coordination has to be relearned as the nerves and muscles wake up. The mind has to focus on the signals sent and received by the brain together with the actual movements of the muscles.

Flexibility

Flexibility is the ability to bend, twist, and turn without breaking. Connective tissue such as ligaments and tendons are not flexible. The muscles, however, are. Muscles should have a lot of elasticity. When you work on flexibility, you should never experience pain. Pain shows that you have reached your limit of elasticity and will cause the opposite effect of what you are trying to accomplish.

Once the muscles get moving, you need to concentrate on stretching and loosening the joints to allow you to reach and bend. Wheelchair users, especially, need to have very flexible movement of their arms and upper bodies in order to overcome the limitations of living in a world designed to accommodate tall, walking people.

Endurance

Endurance is the ability to sustain muscle movements over a period of time. Most textbooks on physical training emphasize strength before endurance. We believe that this should be in reverse order. To develop strength, you must first have the endurance to build the muscles. The Burdenko Method slowly builds endurance by having you perform simple exercises and then increasing the number of repetitions. When the muscles have achieved a proper level of balance, coordination, flexibility, and endurance, then it is time to build speed and strength.

Speed

Speed is the state of moving quickly. Improving speed includes conditioning our reflexes. For normal daily living, you must perform certain functions quickly to avoid injury. For example, wheelchair users must be able to turn their chairs quickly if the situation calls for it. In high levels of training, as in most sports, speed is a measure of performance.

Strength

Strength is the physical power of the muscles. Strength is developed by conditioning the muscles with exercise. It is especially important to develop upper-body strength for mobility in the wheelchair. Muscles that have withered due to underuse as a result of illness, injury, or neglect need to be built up to a healthy working level. You cannot resume your normal functions if the muscles are not properly developed. Beyond rehabilitation lie conditioning and athletic training, where strength is a key factor.

For wheelchair users, it is not necessary to exercise with weights to develop muscle strength. In fact, the use of weights may even be dangerous. Exercise tubing (a stretchable rubber tube) provides a practical, inexpensive, and safe alternative. The resistance from stretching the tubing will provide the same results as weights.

BENEFITS OF THE BURDENKO METHOD

The benefits of the Burdenko Method are manyfold. Its holistic approach not only works to help the body recover from injury, it also helps condition the overall body and enhances one's feelings of well-being and accomplishment.

Physical Conditioning

Wheelchair users need to rely upon their upper-body strength for most of their physical activities. Our conditioning techniques help heal the weakened parts of the body, develop range of motion, and build muscle mass.

Prior to my injury, maintaining balance was an unconscious activity. As any spinal-cord injured person knows, it is embarrassing to fall into your soup at the dinner table whenever you lean forward because your back muscles are weak. The Burdenko Method, therefore, gives special consideration to improving balance, coordination, and flexibility. These now become conscious activities upon which you must focus your efforts. Maintaining body balance and control will soon become second nature. Bending over and sitting upright without the support of the chair helps you resume your normal daily activity.

As the exercise program progresses, you regain strength, endurance, and speed. Simple tasks, like wheeling up inclines and transferring yourself into and out of the wheelchair, which once were exhausting, become effortless. Traveling greater distances in the wheelchair becomes routine. You will be able to get out and around more often. You will have the opportunity to meet and communicate with more people, learn about what is going on in your neighborhood, and make new friends. You will become more engaged in living. This makes life more interesting and generates positive feelings.

Recovery From Injury

Good health takes on greater importance for wheelchair users for obvious reasons. The degree to which you can participate in controlling your life goes hand in hand with your health. Wheelchair users initially find their abilities limited. Society encourages us to accept our limitations and adapt to the surroundings. Many wheelchair users are wrongly told to focus their recovery on coping and re-adjusting.

When you talk to many doctors about rehabilitation, they often offer traditional therapy, modalities, and treatment. We accept these established methods, but the Burdenko Method offers enhancements to traditional rehabilitation. The focus is on waking up and revitalizing the body. It provides the exercises and conditioning you need to gradually return to a state of good health. The degree of health you can achieve is limited only by your ambition and abilities.

The results Dr. Burdenko has achieved have shown time and again that physical limitations can be overcome. Our bodies respond to conditioning. Dr. Burdenko has documented cases of people who have regained the use of their legs and no longer rely on the wheelchair. By constantly attempting to move the muscles, you excite the nerves and recondition the body. At first, there may be no movement. But with persistence, nerves start to tingle, and muscles begin to respond. Then you will begin to see micromovements. With a constant diet of good food, oxygen, exercise, and mental imaging, the body has the opportunity to heal in ways that medicine alone cannot achieve. This is what I am experiencing now!

A Sense of Well-Being and Accomplishment

The Burdenko Method is a maintenance plan for health and life. When you are first born, your body is like a high-performance car. With the proper care and maintenance, it can last and last. Without a proper maintenance program, the car will turn into a piece of junk. Our bodies require the same type of care and maintenance.

Paraplegics can live fulfilling lives whether or not they regain full use of their bodies. However, after an injury, it is easy to fall into a pattern of neglect that causes physical damage and mental distress. A positive attitude is essential to avoid adversity and to get on with life. This program helps you focus on the positive and stay enthusiastic. When used regularly, the techniques of the Burdenko Method will produce results. The thrill and excitement of seeing your legs move again, even just a fraction of an inch, does wonders for your attitude and motivation. Successfully performing exercises that gradually increase in difficulty produces a feeling of accomplishment. It provides inspiration to persevere and to set new goals. You can achieve a level of satisfaction and self-acceptance that adds to the quality of your life.

The Burdenko Method covers a wide range of activities, both mental and physical, based on the philosophy that the body has the power to generate the healing process. After an injury, it is our job to get our bodies into the best possible condition to allow the natural healing process to take place. The Burdenko Method is a program that helps achieve the best results in the shortest amount of time with the least amount of pain.

A major part of recovering from paralysis has to do with stimulating the nerves and reconditioning the muscles. Parts Two and Three of this book cover the land and water exercises specially suited for people with paraplegia and other wheelchair users. It helps wheelchair users improve the quality of their lives by working on developing the muscles to achieve greater balance, coordination, flexibility, endurance, speed, and strength.

Simply stated, the Burdenko Method is an integration and practical application of water and land exercises based on a science to maintain a healthier quality of life and enhance physical performance.

Paul Carney's Story

An unseasonably late snowstorm in May of 1977 had iced over the roads. The day before had been sunny and warm, and I had been playing softball. I had just finished my first semester at college and was looking forward to the summer. As I was driving that day, my car skidded on the ice, and I crashed into the wall. I felt a tingling creep up my toes and legs just before I blacked out.

Later that evening, I overheard the doctors tell my mother that if I survived the night I would be quadriplegic—essentially a vegetable for the rest of my life. I spent the next twenty-two months in the hospital undergoing all kinds of experimental medications and treatments. A side effect of the steroids I had taken caused severe bone damage, and I endured several hip replacements.

This was devastating for me. I had always been athletic and loved to compete. I felt deep down inside that somehow I would beat this thing and find a way to walk again.

After I was out of the hospital for seven years, a friend of mine—Charles Laquidera, a famous Boston disc jockey—recommended that I see Dr. Burdenko. Igor had helped Charles recover from a painful back injury, and Charles said Igor had worked wonders. I met with Igor and discussed my situation. At the time, both of my hips were broken. Even though I had just replaced them, the bones were weak, and I was in so much pain that I didn't realize the extent of the damage. Igor evaluated my situation and explained how he could help me, using a combination of land and water exercises. We agreed to work together to get me into shape.

At first, we worked out with no equipment—just performing basic exercises. Igor would not allow any negative thinking. He was always positive, encouraging me to strive to do better and pushing me to achieve more and more. He shared with me his philosophy of the mind—he told me to believe in myself, that I am what I want to be, and that I can achieve my goals with positive thinking, a competitive drive to win, and hard work. Prior to my accident, I had been a hockey player. As an athlete, I agreed with his intensive conditioning and training methods. Igor was like a start-up button to get me going.

It came time for me to have my hips replaced once again. I decided to get into the best physical condition possible before the operation. I believed that Igor could help me like no other person I had ever met could. I made a commitment to work intensively with Igor for one month. We went to the island of St. Thomas and started working out in earnest.

We began each day at 6 A.M. by swimming in the ocean, followed by vigorous exercises with rubber tubing in the water and on the beach. It was amazing how my body responded to the water exercises. For some moments, I could forget my limitations. Water gave me freedom of movement and relief.

After a healthy breakfast, it was more exercises and a walk with crutches in the sand. In the afternoons, we went to the health club to work out with weights and exercise equipment. Then, back home for more exercises in the pool and supper. After a day of hard work in the water and on the land, Igor would have me undergo relaxation therapy. This was a combination of massage to stimulate the nerves and muscles, massage to relax, and conditioning my mind with positive thinking and visualization of my body healing. Then after a good night's sleep, we'd start the whole process over again.

While we were in St. Thomas, for the first time since my accident, I took a step on the beach by myself without the aid of any crutches. I was so excited! It was a wonderful feeling to be walking. Igor's encouragement to never give up, and to try, try, try had really paid off. When we returned to Boston, my mother saw me walking in the airport terminal and started screaming with joy. Everyone was in tears, but happy tears.

My life has changed since working with Igor. I am pursuing my dreams. Professionally, I am a writer. Personally, I am happily married and just recently had a baby girl (another achievement the doctors said would not be possible).

Scott asked me if I had any words of advice I'd like to share in this book. I say, "Believe in yourself. Don't let even a tiny speck of negative thinking sink in to keep you from achieving your goals."

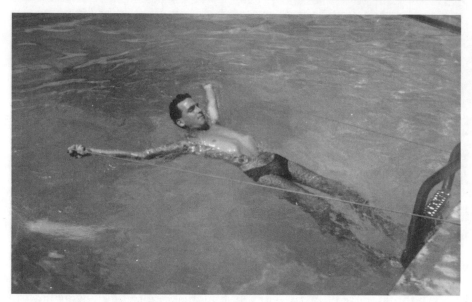

Paul Carney exercising with tubing in the deep end of a swimming pool.

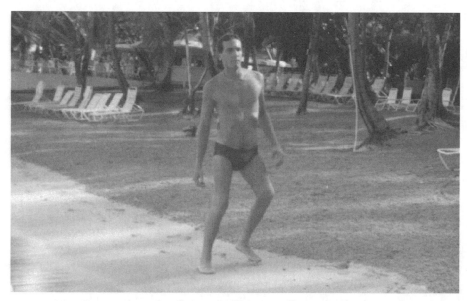

Paul Carney taking his first unassisted steps in seven years.

THREE

The Importance of Using Water to Recover From Injury

Dr. Burdenko's approach to rehabilitation, conditioning, and training relies heavily upon exercising, relaxing, and playing in the water. Recovery from injury in the water occurs faster, more easily, and with less pain than when the same therapy techniques are used on the land.

In this chapter, we will look at how and why water plays such an important part in the Burdenko Method.

THE USE OF WATER AS A MODE OF THERAPY

Many physical therapists and health-care practitioners are coming to appreciate the value of water as a method of therapy. Water has a magical quality that somehow makes rehabilitation seem more like fun than work.

Prior to my accident, I used to enjoy going in the water just for fun. I loved going to the beach and swimming in the ocean, relaxing in a pool, and playing around with my kids in a lake. After my accident, I just figured that I couldn't do those types of things anymore. I had heard of physical therapy in a pool, but my mental image of that was being strapped in a bulky life jacket, with a physical therapist, doing the same rehab exercises that I was used to.

Boy, was I wrong! The first time I got into the water, it was exhilarating. I was able to float and swim in the thin flotation vest without worrying about tipping over. Being in the water again was fun. Dr. Burdenko encouraged me to relax, move around, splash, and enjoy myself. He'd often say, " I want to see you smile." In the water, this was no problem.

So, the first benefit I experienced from the water was psychological. I was able to do something that I did before—and it was fun. If you have any fears or reservations about getting into the water, I encourage you to try it. Wearing some of the new lightweight flotation gear, you do not need to swim to be able to enjoy the water.

In the water, I found that it was much easier to move. My body felt light, and I was free to lean, roll over, or even do a somersault! There was no need to worry about losing my balance or falling. The flotation vest was thin and lightweight, allowing me to move without feeling restricted. I could move and stretch in ways that were impossible on land. And to my surprise, I could do it with much less pain. Moves I could easily make in the water would have hurt too much on land. Unlike land-based exercises, where attempts to move my legs seemed fruitless, in the water the slightest movement of my body could be seen. This ability to see such immediate results really helped my motivation.

So, the water provides a gentle medium in which to work the body. Beginners with weakened or flaccid bodies can use the water, not their muscles, to stretch and relax. Dr. Burdenko's program includes the use of flotation devices, such as the water barbells and kickboard. By simply leaning and swaying in the water, the buoyant effect produced by holding onto this equipment stretches your muscles and moves your joints. This helps reduce muscle tension and improves range of motion and muscle elasticity.

Wheelchair users spend most of their time being sedentary, either sitting or lying down. Pressure sores (decubitus ulcers) are a constant concern. Water provides a medium in which your body can float without the direct pressure of your full weight resting on your legs or back. This aids circulation and gives your body a rest from supporting all your weight.

Being wheelchair-bound, we tend to exercise our bodies less than our walking counterparts do. For those who are not paralyzed, moving the muscles in the lower back, thighs, legs, and feet occurs naturally just when moving around. Standing up, walking, and climbing up and down stairs all provide an opportunity for your body to exercise. This causes your heart to pump harder, providing a fresh supply of oxygen and nourishment throughout your body.

Swimming and exercising in the water have long been used as physical conditioning tools, as evidenced by their acceptance in school athletic programs and Olympic events. Non-wheelchair-users with sore backs are urged to swim as a means of exercise instead of jogging or running. For injuries to the spinal cord, water exercise is a logical choice for physical therapy and conditioning.

After you become accustomed to the water and begin the exercises in this book, you will build up your endurance and be able to enjoy a beneficial workout. Exercising in the water is an easy way to make up for some of the inactivity you experience due to not walking. After a few months, you can build up your stamina. A vigorous exercise session in the water will provide an excellent cardiovascular aerobic workout. Being in the water gives you an opportunity to have some fun and get the exercise your body needs.

A common problem for people with a spinal-cord injury is spasticity (muscle spasms). This can take the form of muscle contractions where the muscles are rigid and hard, or the muscles may contract and relax sporadically, causing the arms or legs to twitch. A water workout provides relief from spasticity for many people. The muscles get exercised in the water and then have a chance to relax.

When you float in the water wearing a flotation vest or belt, your body position is vertical. You stand upright. This is the natural functioning position for humans. Wheelchair users are encouraged to stand erect as much as possible on land through the use of braces, parallel bars, and other equipment. Manufacturers make special wheelchairs and equipment that allow you to strap in and stand up. Standing aids in digestion, bladder function, circulation, and the maintenance of bone strength and muscle tone. The simple act of relaxing in the water upright in your flotation vest has a healthy effect on the body. It is also one of the best positions for support. Floating, supported by the flotation vest, you can relax all your muscles. The weight of your body pulls down on your muscles, and the flotation vest pulls you up. This type of stretching creates more room between the joints. It helps stretch the back muscles and creates more space between the vertebrae to prevent nerve compression and increase circulation and flexibility.

In traditional rehabilitation, exercises and activities are performed on land in a clinic, gym, or physical therapy room. Land-based exercises all rely upon the muscles to resist gravity and carry the weight of the body. The body has to constantly exert enough energy to counteract the force of gravity. When water is used as a modality for rehabilitation, it takes less energy to exercise. The force of gravity in the water is one-tenth of that on land. For example, if a person weighs 150 pounds on land, his or her weight in the water is about 15 pounds.

People feel less pain and are more comfortable in the water. It is our understanding that this occurs because the body does not have to fight against the full force of gravity. In this situation, you save a lot of energy. The laws of physics teach that energy can neither be created nor destroyed; however, energy can be changed from one form into another. Where does this energy go that we have saved by working in the water? We believe that the energy is directed toward helping heal the body.

PHYSICAL PROPERTIES OF WATER THAT MAKE IT IDEAL FOR RECONDITIONING

Water has a number of properties that make it an ideal therapeutic environment. These properties make exercise in the water less difficult and painful, while at the same time, providing resistance to increase the effectiveness of water workouts.

Relative Density

Density is the mass per unit volume of a substance. Relative density is the ratio of the mass of an object to the mass of an equal volume of liquid at standard temperature and pressure.

Relative density determines whether or not an object sinks in water. Simply stated, if an object is denser than water it will sink. With your lungs inflated, your body weighs less than an equal volume of water, meaning it has a low relative density. In other words, you float. When your lungs are deflated, your body weighs more than the water it displaces, meaning it has a higher relative density— i.e., you sink.

Muscle tissue is denser than fat. People who are lean and muscular, therefore, have a higher relative density than those who are not. Men tend to have more muscle mass than women, due to the biological design of their bodies.

Parts of the body that have been swollen after an injury or due to edema (chronic swelling) retain fluid. The fluid is lighter than muscle tissue, giving those parts of the body a low relative density, and they tend to float. Therefore, it takes less effort to raise your extremities (arms and legs) than it does to lower them in the water if they are weak or swollen.

Parts of the body that are limp or paralyzed may experience atrophy—the muscles wither due to lack of exercise. In my case, since I am paraplegic, this has occurred in my legs. With less muscle mass, my legs are relatively lighter.

Buoyancy

Buoyancy is the upward thrust that a fluid exerts on an object less dense than itself. Archimedes, a Greek mathematician, described this force in what has become known as Archimedes' Principle: When a body is fully or partially immersed in a fluid at rest, it experiences an upward thrust equal to the weight of the fluid displaced.

We have established that the human body weighs less than an equal volume of water (when the lungs are inflated). So what keeps buoyancy from pushing us up entirely out of the water? As I am sure you probably have guessed, the answer is gravity. The gravitational force of the earth is trying to pull us down, while buoyancy is trying to push us up. These two forces are constantly opposing each other, and they are in equilibrium when you float partially immersed. In the vertical position, you reach this point when about 90 percent of your body is immersed, with the water up to your neck level.

Buoyancy has a wonderful therapeutic effect on the human body. It can be used to assist or resist movement.

As an assist, buoyancy counteracts the force of gravity, letting your body experience the feeling of weightlessness. The buoyant effect of water puts less strain on the muscles and joints, making it significantly easier to move underwater. This helps you relax and exercise with less pain. This is particularly valuable when attempting to move parts of your body that are stiff or weak, or that have been paralyzed. It takes less effort to see the results.

As a resistance, buoyancy adds difficulty to exercising with flotation devices when pushing or holding the devices underwater. This becomes important for making exercises more challenging as your strength increases.

Hydrostatic Pressure

Everyone knows that if a submarine goes too deep in the ocean, the pressure will cause it to implode. This force is called hydrostatic pressure. This property of water is described in Pascal's Law: Fluid pressure is exerted equally on all surface areas of an immersed body at rest at a given depth.

In laymen's terms, this means that when you are in the water, you feel pressure pushing against your entire body. This hydrostatic pressure has a therapeutic effect in that it helps to increase circulation. It keeps blood from pooling in your arms and legs when low in the water. It also helps increase circulation in areas of your body that are swollen. I have edema in my feet, so being in the water is like wearing a pair of compression stockings, which my medical doctor always recommends.

Hydrostatic pressure makes it harder to breathe when your body is in the water. Although you may not be consciously aware that this is happening, the muscles in your lungs have to work harder to inhale the same volume of air that you would have breathed on the land. So, breathing with the trunk of your body immersed in the water is a form of exercise.

Hydrostatic pressure also helps return the blood to the heart. This will cause your heart to work more efficiently under less pressure. Your pulse and heart rate will go down as a result.

Fluid Resistance

Fluid resistance is the force that tends to oppose or retard the motion of an object through a fluid. The fluid resistance of water is caused by friction and by the clinging action of water molecules to the object. In simple terms, when you move through the water, you have to push your way through all that thick stuff, and it slows you down. The physical properties that explain this are viscosity, adhesion, and cohesion.

Viscosity is the degree to which a fluid resists flow under an applied force. This resistance is caused by the friction your body makes as you move through the water molecules. Cohesion is the attraction of dissimilar molecules. Water molecules actually stick to your body. Adhesion is the attraction between dissimilar molecules. Water molecules tend to stick together, making it difficult to push your way through them.

Fluid resistance is beneficial for water therapy in two ways—It supports and resists movement. As a support, water helps to hold you in position. This means that you won't fall over when you lean or go off balance. As a resistance, water impedes your motion. This added resistance causes your movements through the water to be much slower than in the air. This gives you time to counteract your movements, and it greatly reduces the chance of injury.

One of the first conditions to develop through use of the Burdenko Method is balance. The wonderful fluid resistance of water makes it an ideal place to perform balancing exercises. The water is very forgiving and allows you time to react and relearn how to maintain proper balance in a gentle environment.

Turbulence

Part of the fun of being in the water is splashing, making waves, and hearing the water make that whooshing noise. This is all a result of turbulence. Turbulent flow is the random motion of the water as it moves at changing speeds and pressures, caused by some disturbance.

As you move through the water, pressure builds up in front making waves. At the same time, pressure drops behind, creating a drag that swirls the water in a rotary motion. The combination of these differences in pressure creates the turbulence.

Turbulence provides therapeutic effects in the form of massage and resistance. The swirling and pressure of the water on your body caused by the turbulence act like a gentle massage. This helps increase circulation and reduce pain. Your peripheral nerves are overloaded with the sensation of water all over your skin. This overloading causes the brain to ignore some of the other signals your body is sending (like pain), making the massage feel good.

Turbulence is the main source of resistance that helps exercise the muscles during a water workout. You can vary the resistance by changing the speed, direction, and streamlined effect of your motions. The use of devices like floats and hydrostatic cuffs will reduce the streamlined effect and create more turbulence. This will add resistance as you increase the difficulty of your exercises.

Water therapy is quite beneficial as a means of rehabilitation. It provides a fun way to relax and exercise, putting less stress on the body. You can take advantage of the support and resistance offered by the physical characteristics of water. More than any other modality, water offers the best medium in which to exercise and stimulate paralyzed nerves.

Bob McKenna's Story

In June of 1987, at the age of 23, I fell from a fifth-story balcony. I broke my fifth and sixth cervical vertebrae (C-5 and C-6), which left me paralyzed from the neck down. Fortunately, my father, grandfather, and brother are all doctors. Since they were in the business, they were able to locate the best medical services for me. I was treated at the Boston University hospital, where the doctors fused my neck bones together in a delicate operation that helped save my life. I spent the next six months in the hospital's rehabilitation unit.

In October, I left the hospital. At that point, I needed a personal attendant. I could not roll over, get dressed, get out of bed, or do any preparation by myself. Just maintaining my balance was difficult. I continued to be an outpatient at the Boston University Hospital rehabilitation unit. My rehabilitation program consisted of doing some controlled exercises on a mat for range of motion and to gain some basic strength. My physical therapists talked about my future in terms of ramps and adjusting to life in a wheelchair. I was very frustrated and depressed and did not know what to do with the rest of my life.

My family never gave up hope and continued to search for the best way for me to continue my rehabilitation. My father learned of Dr. Burdenko's work and made arrangements for us to meet. Dr. Burdenko analyzed and evaluated my situation in a way that had not been done before. He expressed an incredible interest in what my body had gone through. For the first time, unlike other rehabilitation specialists, Igor said to me when I couldn't move a muscle, "I understand that you cannot move, but I want you to visualize the movement, thinking about moving it. Even if it doesn't move, I want you to bring it through the motion in your mind." This made a lot of sense to me. I felt that there was movement within my body, even though it couldn't be seen, felt, or even picked up with biofeedback. So Igor's encouragement to visualize the motion was an incredibly powerful tool to me, and in the following months became a primary factor in my reconditioning.

Igor treated me as an athlete in training who wanted to be his personal best. This was unlike traditional therapists who treated me as a patient, or at best a client who was labeled as quadriplegic. I never liked that. I was a young man who had an injury and who wanted to recover from that injury. I did not want to be labeled by some medical term. Igor would never even consider doing something like that. He gave me an incredible amount of respect, which is what I was looking for. This was the type of person I wanted to work with.

We began work that winter. I started with some basic balance exercises on the edge of my seat, trying to strengthen my torso. We also did some floor exercises and worked with exercise tubing, using that as a strengthening tool in different motions. This was to create some torso balance and upper-body strength to prepare me for the pool. Igor said it would be easier to exercise in the water; but that was hard to imagine.

In the spring of 1988, I got into the pool for the first time. Igor and I worked on getting some basic balance, trying to keep my head above water. The freedom of being in the pool was absolutely exhilarating! I just came alive in the water. I felt very comfortable in the pool, being supported and suspended by the water. I wasn't stiff and tight because I wasn't afraid I was going to fall. Igor told me that I was free to make my legs move in any direction. Unlike on land, in the water I had the feeling that I could move. We worked together like sparring partners for five to six days a week in the water. Igor kept me incredibly busy with homework exercises and positions that I practiced religiously three or four times a day. It was like a dream. I actually was able to start moving with maybe just a quiver or a slight movement one way or the other. I became aware of movement in the water that I was unable to instigate on land. So all of this was incredibly encouraging—to actually see my body move and to take it to another level from just feeling it inside me. It really gave me a great mental outlook because the injury had been so overwhelming. To see some progress, to feel good and to have somebody like Igor so focused wanting the best for me, all of these made for a great solution.

As part of my reconditioning, Igor had me work with a massage therapist. As I was being massaged I was encouraged to visualize the movement of my body. As my legs were carried through a range of motion, I was instructed to concentrate as if I were instigating the movement—totally controlling it. As my muscles were being massaged, I focused on sending a positive energy and messages of healing, fluidity, and nerve function.

Another important aspect of his program was nutrition. When I was eating, Igor had me focus on introducing the healthiest building blocks for recovery into my body. I ate foods that were very nutritious and high in fiber. I drank water and other fluids that were nutritious and cleansing. He wanted me to eat foods as a fuel, to give my body energy to strengthen myself.

So Dr. Burdenko introduced me to a new, very positive way of recovering. It was a participatory method of recovery. Nothing was working on me. I was doing the work, and he was assisting me. I was totally focused on my body, concentrating on doing whatever was best.

At the end of the summer, my whole outlook had changed. I felt more energy when I woke up in the morning and throughout the day. That was exhilarating psychologically! Also, it was inspiring to have met such a quality person as Dr. Burdenko and his professional team. I had a new feeling of energy, possibilities, and potential.

In the fall, I returned to school to obtain my degree. Igor was very encouraging. He believes that it is just as important to develop the mind as it is to develop the body. It was good for me to focus on my studies and take a break from the intensive work we did during the summer.

When the next spring came around, I had completed my college degree, and I went back to work with Dr. Burdenko. We worked in the deep end with floatation devices. We spent a great deal of time stimulating and moving my legs. Igor kept instructing me to focus on moving my legs, always visualizing putting them through the movement of running, lifting, and extending.

One day, we were doing my exercises in the pool. Igor was instructing me to concentrate on visualization, and my right leg started to move in a running motion. I couldn't believe it. I started crying, I was so thrilled. Whether we had created a new way for the nerve to communicate, or whether it was persistence, or whatever it was, the leg started moving. Things just took off from there.

I would stand on the bottom, shoulder-deep in the water holding onto floatation barbells. Slowly, I would move up the incline into the shallow end, usually losing my balance and falling over. By the end of the summer, I could actually walk without the barbells and stand in the shallow end. It was spectacular! I remember Igor saying then that thousands of steps in the water were equal to a few steps on the land.

My family never gave up hope, but they really didn't think I would ever walk again. When they came to the pool and saw me walk in the water, they couldn't believe their eyes. It was like a miracle.

So this is how it happened working with Dr. Burdenko. It was through being healthy, working hard, exercising regularly, stimulating the body, looking for new potential. Exercising in the water was enjoyable, which made recovery possible. Weaker muscles that had atrophied could express themselves easier in the water where there was less gravity forcing the leg down or restricting it in any way. Before, when I was in the rehab unit exercising on the mat, it was miserable. I was limited in the direction that my legs might be able to move. It wasn't something you look forward to doing every day. I would intentionally or sometimes unintentionally try to find ways of getting out of it. In the water, I could see the results, which was encouraging and helped to make it an enjoyable experience.

In the two years that I worked with Dr. Burdenko, I went from being confined to my wheelchair and feeling very awkward to walking in the shallow end of a pool. To me this was a virtual recovery. Since then, I have been able to continue my rehabilitation, and today I walk on land with only the support of ankle braces and crutches. I have a fully independent life. I live by myself, work, study, and basically do everything I want. Through Igor I feel I have achieved this. With him I believe there are possibilities that even I haven't thought of yet.

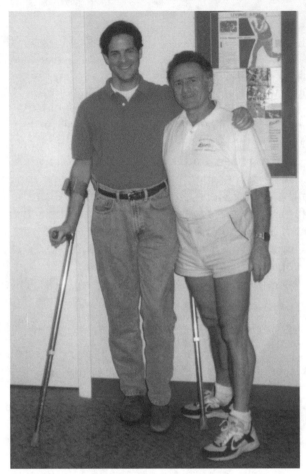

Bob McKenna standing with Dr. Burdenko.

FOUR

Diet Therapy

Good nutrition does not mean going on a diet. To maintain good health, you don't need a diet—you need information. Diets are for when you are sick or recovering from injury. A medical diet is designed for special internal, external, or chronic problems. There is a clear distinction between medical diets and eating nutritionally to maintain good health. When you understand the importance of giving your body the essential food and fluids it needs to function efficiently, choosing what and how to eat become intelligent and enjoyable decisions.

This chapter contains some general guidelines that I learned from Dr. Burdenko and that have proven to be effective. However, it needs to be made clear that your food and liquid intake must be modified according to your goals and your level of disability. I recommend that you consult with a professional nutritionist to help analyze your eating habits and ensure your body is getting the fuel it needs.

As a rule, diets should not be used to control weight. Weight control can be achieved through a lifestyle of eating intelligently and exercising. A weight-loss diet is a short-term fix using specific foods and liquids. That is why most people regain weight in the months following a diet. The short-term diet did not change the eating habits that led to being overweight in the first place.

MY EATING EXPERIENCE

I could have avoided several months of physical and mental anguish after my accident if a professional nutritionist had evaluated my condition. I was hospitalized for about five months. The typical patient at my rehab hospital was elderly and recovering from a stroke, hip replacement, some type of mental disorder, or cancer. The hospital food catered to their tastes (not necessarily to their needs).

Hospital meals were served three times a day. The lunch and supper meals were often interchangeable. So a typical evening meal was:

- Salad: a very small dish of lettuce, a hard wedge of tomato, and some shredded carrot, with plenty of salad dressing.

- Main course: soft, overcooked vegetables, potatoes, or rice, some form of beef or chicken that was usually covered in gravy, and a roll with plenty of butter and jam.

- Dessert: a choice of Jell-O or cake with frosting and ice cream.

- Beverage: always coffee, with a choice of other liquids.

It does not take a nutritional expert to know that these were not healthy meals to eat on a regular basis. I was in several different hospitals during my recovery, and the quality of the meals varied greatly. But even so, I was never visited by a nutritionist who was concerned with how my recovery was affected by what or how I ate. For the most part, even though some nutritional foods were offered, I was able to order just about anything I wanted, regardless of the effect it had on my health.

Initially after my accident, I had lost so much weight that my "special" diet included drinking one or two fortified milkshakes a day with my meals. I was encouraged to put on weight, and was offered plenty of ice cream and other fattening foods.

Coincidentally, the entire five months that I was hospitalized, I was constipated and had to take massive doses of laxatives. This was a great concern for me, and I had several consultations with different doctors. The head of the gastrointestinal department of one of the hospitals I stayed in finally suggested that I consider having a colostomy bag surgically attached. I refused to have the operation. It never occurred to any of the many doctors who reviewed my case that perhaps I needed to alter my diet.

When I was released from the hospital, my wife immediately changed my meals to include high-fiber, low-fat foods. I had plenty of vegetables served fresh or lightly steamed. Milkshakes were replaced with fruit juice. Red meat was replaced with chicken and fish. Cake and frosting was replaced with fresh fruit. My wife prepared wonderful soups from fresh vegetables and herbs. Within a few weeks, my digestive system started to work on its own, and I threw all the laxatives away. This change in my eating habits played a significant role in correcting a serious medical problem that had plagued me for months.

So, I cannot stress enough the importance of good nutrition. After an injury, everything changes: your mobility, lifestyle, and habits; and so, too, should your nutrition. Not only do the quality of the food and the way it is prepared matter, but the time of day you eat, the way you eat, food portion sizes, and eating habits are also important and should be reevaluated and adjusted. With the proper eating habits, you can help control your weight, prevent mood swings, keep wastes and toxins from accumulating in your body, and return to a good state of health.

DEVELOP PROPER EATING HABITS

It was about a year after my accident that I met Dr. Burdenko. On our first meeting, he made an assessment of my physical condition and introduced me to his method of rehabilitation. From the very beginning, he stressed the importance of proper nutrition in helping the body to heal itself. The rest of the information that appears in this chapter I learned from him and his daughter Nelle, who is a nutritionist.

How You Eat

Your body responds well to a regimen. You should develop a routine; wake up, go to bed, and eat meals at the same time day after day to make your body work as a clock.

As a general rule, meals should be eaten hot, warm, or at room temperature—not cold—or with hot liquids. This warms the stomach and helps in getting nutrients into the bloodstream and the body.

It is better to eat several small meals (about four or five) throughout the day than to have three big meals. This keeps your energy level up throughout the day, and it prevents your digestive system from being overworked. Additionally, several small meals will help satisfy your hunger since you will eat more often, even though you are not eating a larger quantity.

Here are some guidelines for developing proper eating habits:

- Do not overemphasize any specific type of food in your diet. Eat a little bit of everything.

- Eat slowly and chew your food thoroughly.

- Do not overeat. Stop eating before you feel full.

- Start your day with a hot breakfast.

- Try having soup with your lunch instead of a beverage, and make lunch the biggest meal of the day.

- Your evening meal (supper) should be lighter than your lunch.

- The last meal of the day should be eaten three to four hours before your bedtime.

- Maintain your optimal weight.

- Before eating, wash your hands with soap—bacteria tends to build up on your palms.

- Make sure your vegetables are fresh and clean. Wash them with warm water before eating.

- Don't combine dairy products and fish, dairy products and meats, or dairy products and vegetables in the same meal. Different digestive enzymes are required to process different types of food, and these different enzymes are not all available at the same time.

- Remove the skin from fish and poultry because skin contains lots of toxins and is a rich source of fats.

- Swallow in small portions. This adds more saliva to each portion. The increased moisture added to swallowed food helps digest it.

- Focus on your food while eating—do not read or watch television (keep your mind and body functioning together).

- Plan your cooking, eating, and snacking ahead of time.

- Read food labels—not only the ingredients, but also the expiration date.

- When you get hungry between meals, eat fresh or dried fruits and vegetables. Hunger affects your attitude. When you are hungry, you usually don't smile, and you may develop a negative attitude.

- Monitor your blood pressure and cholesterol levels.

What You Eat

To make your body work efficiently, the food in your diet must be varied, balanced, and eaten in moderate quantities. It is important to keep all the food groups in mind when planning your diet. Every day, your diet should include something from each of these groups: breads and grains; fruits and vegetables; milk and dairy products; and meats, poultry, and fish. You should eat at least five different fruits and vegetables every day.

Here are some guidelines on what to eat:

- Buy good quality fresh, frozen, or dried foods from reputable sources.

- Try to avoid foods from cans—there may be lots of preservatives, sodium, or heavy syrup in them.

- Balance your vitamin and mineral intake.

- Squeeze lemon on salads, fish, meats, and poultry to help prevent bacterial growth.

- Eat one to two cloves of raw garlic twice a week to disinfect your digestive tract.

- Eat watermelon and cucumbers to stimulate kidney function and urination.

- Substitute table sugar with honey (which is also an antiseptic), maple syrup, and dried fruits.

- Eat lots of deep orange and yellow fruits. The beta-carotene and fructose will help balance your energy level.

- Eat calcium-containing products, like cottage cheese and yogurt, to prevent osteoporosis and to help in removing toxins from your body.

- Plan your menu to include foods with plenty of vitamins and minerals.

- Drink plenty of fluids.

Vitamins and Minerals

Enzymes are needed as catalysts for every bodily process. Without enzymes, our bodies could not function. Likewise, enzymes could not function without vitamins. Vitamins ("vita" means life) are called coenzymes. We do not need them in megadoses, but we need the whole spectrum of them every day. Food should be your primary source of vitamins and minerals; however, for those who do not take in adequate nutrients in their diets, supplementation is a viable means of obtaining the vitamins and minerals necessary for health and recovery. Of particular importance to those of us recovering from nerve damage are the vitamins and minerals responsible for nerve functions: vitamins B_1, B_3, B_5, and B_6 and the minerals calcium, phosphorus, and copper. See Table 4.1 below for a list of some of the vitamins and minerals so vital to nerve function.

Fats

There is a lot of media hype these days on television and in magazines about maintaining a low-fat diet (there's that word diet again). We agree that you should not eat fat in excess. However, be careful not to eliminate fat from your diet entirely. Fat serves a purpose:

- It surrounds your internal organs and acts as a cushion.

- It helps regulate your body temperature (it is like insulation in your house).

- It is needed by your hormones.

So, fat should not be eliminated from your food intake but taken in moderation.

TABLE 4.1. VITAMINS AND MINERALS RESPONSIBLE FOR NERVE FUNCTIONS.

Nutrient	Food Sources
Vitamin B_1 (thiamin)	Pork, fortified grains and cereals, seafood.
Vitamin B_3 (niacin or nicotinic acid)	Poultry and seafood, seeds and nuts, or potatoes, fortified whole grains and cereals.
Vitamin B_5 (pantothenic acid)	Almost all plant and animal foods. Also manufactured by intestinal bacteria.
Vitamin B_6 (pyridoxine)	Meats, fish, and poultry; grains and cereals; spinach; sweet potatoes; white potatoes; bananas; prunes; watermelon.
Calcium	Milk and milk products, canned salmon (with bones), oysters, broccoli, tofu.
Phosphorus	Dairy products and egg yolks; meat, poultry, and fish; legumes.
Copper	Lobster, organ meats, nuts, dried peas, beans, prunes, barley.

Typical Recommended Menu

The following is an example of a typical menu for one day:

Breakfast: Hot cereal with dried fruits or honey, herbal tea.

Lunch: Split-pea soup, scallops with rice and salad, tea.

Afternoon Snack: Fresh strawberries, toast, herbal tea.

Supper: Squash with lemon, whole-wheat crackers with jam, tea.

Liquid Intake

Your body is 80-percent liquid. It needs an ongoing supply of fluids for metabolism and digestion, as well as for the life and function of your body's cells. However, it is our belief that too much liquid can be harmful to your heart. By increasing your blood volume, you exhaust your heart pump. When you do not take in enough liquid, the balance of your biochemical reactions shifts, causing everything to shrink. (Picture flowers without water or grass without rain.) Without liquids to carry off the byproducts of digestion, your body will accumulate wastes. So, drink plenty of fluids to stimulate urination and wash these toxins away; however, monitor your liquid intake carefully to maintain the fine natural balance your body requires.

Here are some guidelines to develop good liquid intake habits:

- While it is recommended that the average healthy individual drink eight glasses of water per day, those who are wheelchair-bound need only drink five to six 8-ounce glasses of water per day, due to their limited movement.

- Drink plenty of water that is clean and pure. (Your tap water may be heavily chlorinated or have residual chemicals. In this case, drink distilled water.)

- Try to avoid drinks with caffeine, sodium, or high amounts of sugar.

- Drink hot tea after every meal to dissolve fats and speed up the digestive process.

- Drink fruit juices as sources of fluids and vitamins.

- Reduce your liquid intake two to four hours before you go to bed so that you do not interrupt your sleep with bathroom trips.

- Limit your use of alcoholic beverages. Excessive alcohol affects your attitude as well as your liver.

Stimulating Your Digestive Tract

Eat plenty of roughage (fiber) to stimulate your bowel movements in order to eliminate the toxins from your systems. Fresh and dried fruits and vegetables are good sources of fiber. Grains work like sandpaper to clean the lining of your stomach and intestines. Contract and relax your abdominal muscles in a wavelike motion, and change the position of your body from time to time while you lie down or sit to stimulate peristalsis. Maintaining a regimen of defecating at the same time each day helps the digestive system function smoothly.

Choose a good diet therapist, just as you would choose a good physician. Honor your body and supply it with the proper building blocks it needs to be healthy. I have learned that eating intelligently is not stressful like dieting. Once you begin eating nutritionally, I am sure you will notice that it becomes enjoyable. Good nutrition should be a lifetime commitment. Your body deserves the best! Dr. Burdenko frequently reminds me that it is just as important to eat the right foods and drink the proper liquids as it is to exercise the mind and body. Proper nutrition is part of conditioning the whole body.

FIVE

Conditioning Principles and Techniques

A significant portion of this book is dedicated to exercises. Paying attention to how you prepare for an exercise session is just as important as what you do during and after the exercises. I am not talking about a warm-up and cool-down period—these are parts of the exercises themselves. I am talking about the techniques you use to get the most benefit from the exercise session both physically and mentally.

These principles and techniques that you will use to condition your body apply to all exercises. Part of Dr. Burdenko's philosophy is that you work on conditioning the whole body, not just the specific area that has been injured or the particular muscles being exercised at the moment. As you will see, it is important to incorporate proper techniques such as breathing, relaxing, and acquiring the proper mindset into all exercises sessions. I recommend that you review these conditioning principles and techniques from time to time to make sure you incorporate all of them into your daily routine.

PHYSICAL CONDITIONING

There are many aspects to physical conditioning. In addition to the exercises themselves, it is important that you pay attention to shaking the body awake before the exercises; proper breathing, body awareness, and relaxation while performing the exercises; and the benefits of massage before and after exercising.

Shaking

Shaking is the technique we use to wake up the body for exercise, to relax, and to improve circulation to the muscles during training and to aid in recovery from each workout. It's a simple but effective method that maximizes the benefits of this program.

During the warm-up phase of exercise, shaking increases the temperature in the tissues and loosens tight muscles and joints. Loose, relaxed muscles function more efficiently, maximizing the benefits of exercise.

While exercising, the demand for oxygen in the muscles is high. Blood flows vigorously through the circulatory system, delivering the much needed oxygen. When the exercise stops, the blood tends to pool in the muscles, where it is not needed. Shaking after exercising is a technique to help the muscles relax and to improve the circulation. So, perform shaking between exercises and during cool-down periods.

Ideally, shaking should be done with the arms and legs. (See Figure 5.1, below.) Depending upon your level of functioning, you may be limited, as I am, to shaking only your arms. If this is the case, follow these directions for shaking:

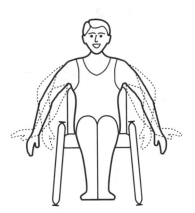

- Sit erect with your arms down at your sides.

- Gently begin by shaking your arms.

- Let your wrists and hands stay loose and relaxed.

- Now shake more vigorously for fifteen to twenty seconds.

- Repeat the process. Get loose!

- Next move your arms to your sides, overhead, out in front of you, or behind you and begin shaking again.

Figure 5.1. Shaking.

Then, if you have use of your legs, stretch them, and rest your heels on the floor. Bend each knee alternately. You can also lift each leg and shake it. Make sure your entire body is relaxed while doing this. Always start slowly and progressively move faster and faster.

Proper Breathing

Breathing is going to take on new meaning in your life. No longer will breathing be an absent-minded function. Muscle growth and nerve-damage repair require an abundant supply of oxygen that deep breathing can provide.

All body metabolism ultimately relies on oxygen consumption. If you spent any time in a hospital after a serious injury, you probably received oxygen to aid in your recovery. Any body movement or muscular activity lasting more than a minute and a half requires a new supply of energy to keep the muscles functioning. This energy is obtained from a process called cellular oxidation, whereby oxygen is used to break down food (carbohydrates, fats, or proteins) providing energy to the muscles. As you build strength and endurance, your muscles will require more and more oxygen. Indeed, one measure of physical fitness is the maximum rate at which an individual can consume oxygen.

When you inhale, you do not use your lungs to full capacity, as there is always air left inside the lungs after exhaling. To get as much oxygen as possible into your system, you must perform deep breathing exercises. This can be done by intentionally lifting the diaphragm in the chest, breathing in and blowing out large volumes of air. It can also be done automatically through exercise. When we exercise, the muscles demand oxygen, sending a signal to the brain that stimulates an increase in the rate of breathing. The brain also activates three additional muscles in the chest to expand the lungs and increase their capacity. As the lungs are filled, the air pressure inside increases. This is like blowing up a balloon and feeling the air push out against the sides of the balloon. It creates a difference in pressure that forces the oxygen from the lungs into the bloodstream.

There are many techniques for deep breathing. We recommend the following technique because we find it to be the most effective and least painful and easy to learn. You should perform breathing exercises in the fresh air. Outdoors is the best place to be, unless the air quality is poor.

- Begin by inhaling through your nose. This filters and warms the air as it enters into your lungs.

- Lift your chest as you inhale, raising the diaphragm. Let your chest expand, filling up all the chambers in your lungs. (See Figure 5.2 on page 50.)

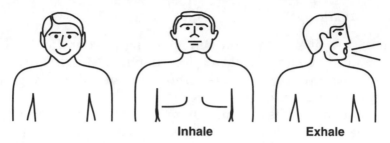

Figure 5.2. Proper breathing action.

- Purse your lips together and blow the air out through the small hole between your lips (like blowing out a candle). Push hard.

You can practice stretching and exercising your neck as you breathe. Each time you exhale, turn your head in a different direction: left, right, forward, up, and down.

Breathing is equally important for cleansing the system. The body needs to expel carbon dioxide carried by the blood into the lungs and remove toxins and wastes through the lymph system. Deep breathing is the force that drives these purging mechanisms. Make deep breathing a daily priority.

Body Awareness

Body awareness is the use of your senses to control the position of your body while exercising. It includes maintaining balance, knowing where your center of gravity is located, and paying attention to the proper positioning of each part of your body. While exercising, body awareness includes control of your breathing. You should be conscious of breathing throughout the exercise: avoid holding your breath. Inhale when your chest is lifted or your extremities are extended, and exhale when your chest is lowered or your extremities are retracted. Whenever you exercise, you should practice maintaining body awareness. This means that you should concentrate on performing the exercises correctly. Many athletes exercise in front of mirrors to observe their movements for this reason.

As you exercise, it is useful to have your trainer or an assistant watch and let you know when your balance is not right, when you are not erect, or if your elbows drop when they are supposed to be at shoulder level, etc. I often think that I am really doing a great job on my exercises until Igor watches me and gives me the feedback that I need to make corrections.

It is especially difficult to see how you are doing when in the water. I have been surprised many times when I looked down to see what my legs were doing. Sometimes, they actually go where my mind is visualizing them to be. Regaining body awareness is especially important when recovering from injury, a time when you have limited sensations.

The more feedback you get, the better you will become at maintaining your own body awareness. Make it a conscious effort.

Massage

Massage has been used for centuries as a powerful healing therapy by many different cultures. It is well accepted as a form of treatment and relaxation therapy throughout Europe and the Far East. In Russia, where Dr. Burdenko obtained his Ph.D. in Sports Medicine, massage is one of the strongest modalities used in conditioning and recovering from injuries. Massage can be used in conjunction with other modalities of therapy to relieve pain, muscle soreness, and stress, and to help generate the healing process. I believe that massage will become more accepted in the United States as people grow to understand its benefits and appreciate the results.

There are many types of massage therapy. One element they all have in common is that the therapist touches the patient's body. They may do this with their hands, elbows, knees, or instruments. The power of human touch provides a psychological benefit that cannot be matched by taking medications. You feel cared for in a personal way that creates a feeling of satisfaction and well-being. I believe that this contributes to the power of positive thinking, which is such a strong part of Dr. Burdenko's method in helping the body heal itself. Aside from this, massage offers such direct benefits as muscle relaxation, improved range of motion through stretching of the joints, increased circulation of the blood to deliver oxygen and nutrients to the body, increased circulation of extracellular body fluids to remove waste products, improved body temperature, and relief from tension and stress. All of these benefits contribute to your emotional well-being.

There are several different massage techniques. In Europe, a popular form of massage is known as Swedish massage. It is primarily a modality of stroking and rubbing the body. In the Far East, a different form of massage has developed that involves acupressure and stretching, called shiatsu. I recommend that you experience several of the different techniques. You may prefer one style more than another.

There are four basic types of massage that Dr. Burdenko recommends: general relaxation, sports, selective, and therapeutic. A general relaxation massage is very helpful in relaxing the muscles, reducing tension, and relieving stress. A sports massage is given to reinvigorate the body after the muscles have been thoroughly exercised, and you feel sore or exhausted. A selective massage focuses on a particular part of the body, such as a pulled hamstring. Therapeutic massage is a whole-body massage that reduces pain and increases circulation and is used as treatment for an injury or particular condition.

In most massage techniques, the patient lies still and simply receives the treatment. For people who are paralyzed from a stroke or an accident, Dr. Burdenko uses a therapeutic massage involving a combination of techniques to stimulate muscle and nerve function. It is a participatory massage, where you play an important role in increasing the efficiency of the massage with your imagination, nerve energy, and body energy.

Following an injury, the muscles shrink from inactivity. Nerves act the same way. They get shorter in length and smaller in diameter when they are not used. With Dr. Burdenko's technique, as you are massaged, visualize your nerves, and imagine the sensations passing through them and building bridges across the damaged area. Try to feel the energy going through the muscles and revitalizing them. You should work together with the massage therapist. This is a team approach. As the therapist lifts and manipulates the paralyzed limbs, you have to picture the nerves and muscles being stimulated and relaxed, both of which generate the healing process.

There are a few general guidelines that Dr. Burdenko follows in administering massage that are worth mentioning:

- The environment for the massage should be warm and comfortable. You should feel relaxed and be able to focus your mind on pleasant thoughts, without being disturbed by noises or interruptions.

- Massage should be given at the proper time. A massage should not be given immediately following a meal. If you generate more circulation in one area, you take it away from the stomach, where it is needed to digest the food.

- Massage should always be pleasant. I believe that massage should never cause pain. The type you should receive depends upon your present condition. If you have an injury, the area surrounding the injury (not the injured area itself) should be massaged.

- Massage should always be done in the direction of the lymph nodes—under the armpits, in the groin, and in the neck area just under the jaw—and the heart. The lymph nodes, which remove toxins, act as the body's sewage system. So as you massage, use your hands to stimulate circulation of the blood and removal of toxins through the lymph system.

- The massage should have three distinct phases. Begin with gentle, long stroking and broad circular motions to relax the muscles and increase circulation. The second phase is the main portion of the massage. It is used to stimulate the muscles and nerves, work the joints, carry off waste products, and remove tension. Here, you work the muscles with stronger motions. There are a variety of different techniques that you can use, including pulling, squeezing, kneading, wringing, chopping, pinching, drumming, a rolling motion, and rubbing in a zigzag fashion. The last phase of the massage is similar to the beginning, with gentle stroking and rubbing. This ends the massage, leaving the patient feeling sleepy, stress-free, and fully relaxed.

- Massage of the facial muscles is effective in stress relief. Your face is the center of all emotions. Facial expressions help your body communicate your level of stress and tension. After a facial massage, relax the muscles with a hot compress.

- After a massage, cover your body with a hot, moist towel and wrap your body in blankets as if you were in a cocoon. Lie still for a few minutes. This will help increase circulation and will have a mental and physical therapeutic effect.

I recommend that you get a book on massage and learn the basics. Massage techniques are simple and can be easily followed by you and your family members. As you become more skilled in massage, you work with your hands to increase circulation, relax the muscles, change the muscle tone, and gain relief from stress. People in wheelchairs should undergo massage therapy every day. This will help the body regenerate and heal the damaged tissues. At the same time, you will have a sense that your body is helping to heal itself. You will be able to feel the progress you are making in your recovery.

MENTAL CONDITIONING

I am amazed at the stories Dr. Burdenko tells me about his quadriplegic patients, like Bob McKenna and Paul Carney, who have learned how to walk again, and stories of other physically challenged individuals and handicapped athletes who can now run marathons and compete in sporting events like swimming, sprinting, and shot put. People who had virtually given up on life now have fulfilling careers, have gotten married, and have even had babies. They have healed their paralyzed bodies using Igor's techniques. They refused to let doctors tell them that they'd never walk again, and with sheer determination and will they recovered. If you believe you can accomplish something, you will find that you are capable of achieving goals that were otherwise unobtainable. The human body has no limits. Look at the world records in sporting events now compared with those of just ten years ago.

The human body has incredible powers to heal itself. We have all heard stories of cancer patients who have refused to die and willed themselves to heal, and people who recover from serious illness and even wind up competing and winning in the Olympics, such as Wilma Rudolph. These people have tapped into the power of their minds.

Attitude

Attitude is everything. Some of us are blessed with continued optimism. Others need help in remaining enthusiastic about anything. How we see the world and deal with it influences our behavior. You are what you want to be. If you act discouraged, sad, or angry, people will treat you with pity and sympathy. If you act happy or enthusiastic, you make people feel good, and they are glad to see you. The way you behave is picked up by other people and gets reflected right back at you. Think of your own mind in this same way. If you act happy, you will be happy. If you believe you can get better, you will get better.

When I first began working with Dr. Burdenko, I did not understand how important attitude was. Dr. Burdenko told me I could do things that everyone else said were impossible. When I started believing that, it really changed my attitude and directly affected the effort I put into the program. Now I realize how essential attitude is.

Participate in activities that reinforce a positive attitude. Look into the mirror and smile at yourself. It really works! Smile when you exercise. Do not engage in negative thinking. Listen to tapes of motivational speakers, like Tony Robbins. Look forward to each day as an opportunity to work on your recovery.

Igor often says, "Life is an opportunity to catch positive emotions."

Visualization

Visualization is a powerful tool to use while exercising to wake up your mind and body. It involves picturing whatever your goal may be actually happening. As you attempt to move your legs, even though it may feel like nothing is happening, picture your legs moving in your mind. If you wobble while you work out in the wheelchair, imagine sitting erect. Remember how it used to feel. Think about what muscles are used in sitting erect. Use your mind to stimulate the nerves and muscles that have been damaged or neglected.

Imagine that you see inside your body. As you breathe, visualize the oxygen entering your lungs, passing into the bloodstream, traveling out through the arteries, branching out through the body, leaving the bloodstream, and going right into the neurons (nerve cells). Picture the neurons healing. See them branching out and regenerating. As you work your muscles, picture them taking in the oxygen and nutrients from the blood to revitalize and get strong. See them developing and getting bigger and stronger.

In your mind's eye, picture yourself in good health—walking, running, playing, and back to normal. Keep generating positive signals to help stimulate your body to heal itself. It just may work!

Meditation

Meditation basically involves setting a time aside to relax the body and to focus your thoughts. It is often used as a tool for controlling pain and achieving peace and tranquillity. Meditation allows the mind to overcome the limitations of the body. It is a restful time when you tap into the energy from within.

Many hospitals, schools, and other institutions offer courses in meditation. If you have not had an opportunity to meditate, we recommend that you look into learning more about it.

COMBINING PHYSICAL STIMULATION WITH MENTAL CONDITIONING TO OPTIMIZE REHABILITATION

The preceding section dealt with using the mind as a source for initiating rehabilitation and conditioning. You have learned to use your mind to stimulate your body and send signals out through the body. You can also use your body to stimulate your mind to then send the necessary signals throughout the body. This is done through physical stimulation of the body, which is picked up by the receptors in the nerves and sent back to the brain.

People who have suffered brain damage are encouraged to use this technique of physical stimulation. They keep bombarding the brain with nerve impulses from continued physical stimulation, which helps them regain their senses.

As part of your exercise routine, you should move the paralyzed or weak parts of your body, even if you cannot feel anything. This can be done with the aid of exercise tubing or flotation devices. You can also have an assistant pick up your legs or help you move your arms while you exercise. Massage is an excellent source of physical stimulation for paralysis. The nerves in your extremities will try to transmit those physical sensations back to the brain. Watch closely as your legs are moved by your assistant. Take that visual image and coordinate in your mind how the actual movements should feel.

This combination of physical stimulation and willing your nerves to respond is a powerful technique to help the body heal itself. It is right at the heart of Dr. Burdenko's method, which he uses to help his patients recover from paralysis.

Exercise is an important part of the Burdenko Method. The effectiveness of the exercise routine is greatly affected by the principles and techniques that you use. How you breathe and relax and what you think about all play parts in the whole exercise routine. Especially for people recovering from paralysis, it is important to work on your frame of mind along with the physical activities to stimulate the natural healing process.

Sebastian DeFrancesco's Story

I am a C-5, 6 quadriplegic, meaning that my quadriplegia is the result of injury to the fifth and sixth cervical bones in my neck. This injury resulted from a military jeep accident. I have been in a wheelchair for nineteen years. Following my accident, I have tried to keep myself in good physical condition.

I first met Igor in 1983 when I was in training for the Paralympic Games. Through his expertise in rehabilitation and conditioning, he was able to analyze my situation and provide me with a routine of exercises to improve my balance, flexibility, and endurance. I found Igor to be a person I could trust, who desired to help make me into a better athlete, and who has a lot of passion for what he does. We began doing many different exercises in the wheelchair with rubber tubing. I never liked working with weights, and the tubing provided an easy way to get a thorough workout.

In 1984, Igor accompanied the United States Paralympic team to the Paralympic Games in Stoke Mandville, England. This was the first time that a strength and conditioning trainer had ever assisted members of the United States Paralympic team. His enthusiasm and willingness to help kept him very busy. Many of the wheelchair athletes were eager to work with him and take advantage of his experience and expertise.

When you compete as an athlete in the Paralympic Games, you are placed into a class based on your abilities. After working with Igor, I felt that my training had improved so much that I could compete at a higher level. The level of conditioning that Igor helped me attain in balance and mobility added to my performance for sure and helped me win the silver and bronze medals in table tennis.

I still use the rubber tubing exercises that I learned from Igor. They help keep me in shape today.

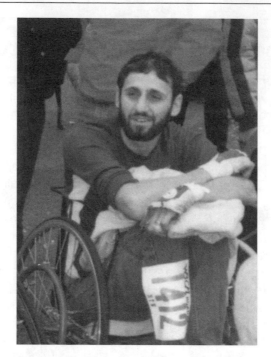

Sebastian DeFrancesco at the 1984
Paralympic Games in Stoke Mandville, England.

SIX

Dealing With Pain and Depression

Pain is a natural occurrence following an injury. Depression is a complicated condition that can result from a variety of different factors. Pain and depression do not necessarily go together. You can be depressed without having any physical pain, and vice versa. I have grouped them together here in this chapter since most people who are paralyzed were in an accident that was painful, and the accident also had a devastating effect on their lives. Under these circumstances, it is quite common to experience some depression. Pain and depression do have one thing in common—they are problems that consume a lot of energy and that distract you from focusing your attention on staying healthy.

Pain is a complicated subject that is not fully understood by physicians and scientists. The treatment of pain is often addressed by administering a medication, without fully understanding why the medications do or do not work. When pain is intense, medications may be appropriate. For long-term health, I believe that it is better to be free of all medications. So my discussion on pain will deal more with why we have pain and how to cope with it.

I am not an expert on depression. I do have personal experience in learning how to deal with paralysis, which, to say the least, was not a happy occasion. I also suffer from chronic pain which often leads to depression for some people. So, I will share the information I learned about depression, in hopes that it will be helpful to you.

TYPES OF PAIN

Pain can occur in different forms—physical and physiological. When I speak of pain, I am referring to physical pain—a specific location on your body that hurts. Most pain is acute, which simply means it is a result of an injury and will diminish and disappear as the injury heals. Long-term pain is called chronic pain.

Acute Pain

Acute pain is a way our bodies send status signals to the brain telling us where we are injured and when we need to rest. Pain from tension tells us when we are distressed. Tingling or burning may be a sign that nerves are regenerating. Pain from exercising is a sign of fatigue that lets us know that we have exerted our muscles to their limits.

Injuries are often accompanied by swelling, which usually causes pain. In the case of spinal-cord injuries, most of the damage to the spinal cord is caused by inflammation that cuts off blood supply to the central nervous system. Pain may also be caused by damaged tissues, sprained muscles, and broken bones. Immediately following an injury, it may be appropriate to receive pain medication to reduce swelling and relieve the intense pain.

You may be fortunate and have little or no pain. For you, a strenuous workout may invigorate and relax. You will need to pace your activity, so as not to overdo. As a general rule, *never work out when you feel pain.* As you begin to exercise, you may experience pain from injuries that have not yet healed and fatigue from muscles that have atrophied. It is important that you realize that these are beneficial pains as you perform the exercises. You need to listen to your body, however, and regulate the amount of exercise you engage in according to your level of pain. Do not surpass your limits. If a particular exercise really hurts, do not continue. There are enough exercises in this book for you to select some that do not cause pain. Be gentle and kind to yourself while you heal, but try to exercise frequently. In some cases, the pain may get worse before it gets better. This is particularly true as nerves regenerate. You may even find yourself looking forward to experiencing these new pains. As injuries heal and muscles develop, it is customary to enjoy a decrease in pain making it worth all the effort it took.

Chronic Pain

In some cases, pain may be chronic, where it serves no useful purpose at all. Chronic pain persists long after an injury has healed. As I mentioned earlier, I have chronic pain. I have not had a day without pain since my accident. Somewhere between 10 and 20 percent of spinal-cord injuries result in some kind of chronic pain. It may be a burning sensation, a feeling of extreme pressure or squeezing, an ache, or a stabbing pain. I experience all of them. I have visited many doctors and specialists looking for someone who could help me, but the medications just don't seem to have any effect. I have tried alternative forms of medication as well. Herbal teas and homeopathic remedies have yet to help. I am just one of those people who have to learn to live with it. I have considered dorsal root nerve surgery to cut or burn the nerves, but this is a serious operation, and in my case, the results are not guaranteed. In the worst case, they may cut some nerves that still function properly.

The advice I was frequently given was to keep busy and ignore the pain. When people would tell me this, my attitude was "Maybe that works for you, but my pain is severe." The pain gets so bad that I have to stop exercising from time to time, but I never give up.

PAIN MANAGEMENT

Pain medications are often prescribed as a treatment for acute and chronic pain; however, these drugs override your body's signals. Additionally, pain medications usually have other side effects and complications. Ultimately, the body builds a tolerance to the medications, and the dosage is increased and increased with lessening results. For long-term health, I believe it is best to be free of all pain medications if at all possible.

When you suffer from severe or prolonged pain, it is usually recommended that you attend some type of pain-control program. Traditionally, these programs fall into two categories. The first is generally referred to as a pain clinic. This is the type of program where you are usually an inpatient at a hospital or health-care institution. The focus of the program is to find the medications or therapy techniques that kill the pain.

The other category is pain management. This is generally an outpatient program for people who have not been able to get rid of their pain. The focus is on learning how to deal with the pain and not let it control your life.

I attended the twelve-week pain-management program at the Deaconess Hospital in Boston. There, I learned that pain can be a vicious cycle. When you are in pain, you feel distressed (unhappy, angry, grouchy, desperate, etc.) When you are distressed, you get tense and your muscles tighten. The tightening of your muscles aggravates the pain, and the cycle starts all over again. Relaxation can help you break out of this cycle. This can be done with biofeedback, relaxation techniques, and meditation. Many of the students at the program would meditate and use visualization to picture their pain as a monster or a fire. They would then envision killing the monster or putting out the fire with ice and would actually experience physical relief from the pain. My attempts at meditation were not so successful, but it worked wonders for some. Another key part of the program was to work on improving our attitudes. Do not engage in negative thinking or self put-downs. Do not associate with people who do. Concentrate on doing things that are fun and give meaning to your life. Don't sit around all day feeling sorry for yourself. Get busy and participate in life. (This reminds me of Igor's 5 Fs: Future, Fitness, Fun, Family, and Friends—Fantastic!) My pain may not be any better, but I've learned to live with it for now.

A change of pace helps to keep your mind occupied and distract your thoughts from the pain. Dr. Burdenko encourages me to change my routine all the time. Exercise in different locations. Change the rooms in which you work, eat, and relax. Rearrange your routine. Perform relaxation techniques at different times. Visualize walking and feeling good. Meet with friends and family regularly, and enjoy their company.

Igor wanted me to stop thinking about my pain, so he gave me the project of writing this book. Many times, when the pain was so bad that I could hardly stand it, I would get up and start working on this book. I'd get so involved that I truly didn't even think about the pain. So, it is really true. If you get your mind focused on something important or an interesting issue, it takes your mind off the pain. I find that the more complex the issue, the more I have to concentrate, and the longer I can distract my thoughts from the pain.

The program described in this book gives you something to look forward to each day. The exercises, especially those designed to stimulate the damaged nerves, require a great deal of concentration. Stay focused on getting better!

Most people find that being in the water is the best way to relax. Without having to resist the full force of gravity, the muscles can go limp. You can float in the warm, comfortable water, forget about your problems, and let stress drift away. This is one reason that many people feel less pain in the water.

DEPRESSION

Being paralyzed or wheelchair-bound is a difficult situation with which to deal. This is especially true right after an accident, when the realization of how it may affect your life becomes overwhelming. It is quite normal to feel bad and be depressed. Depression can be brought on by a number of factors, including despair, isolation, loss of function (paralysis), a chemical imbalance, and stress.

There is a difference between feeling depressed and being clinically depressed, which requires medical or psychological care. Sometimes, the person suffering from depression does not even realize that he or she is suffering from the disorder. Symptoms generally develop gradually over a period of weeks. A depressed person may appear sad and irritable. Eating and sleeping patterns are usually affected. A depressed person generally becomes withdrawn, loses interest in activities he or she once enjoyed, and has little or no sexual desire. Fortunately, I was not clinically depressed. In extreme cases of despair, when a person withdraws into a shell or is contemplating suicide, medical attention is required.

Typical Causes of Depression Following an Accident

It is normal for depression to accompany a bad accident, especially one so serious that it causes you to need a wheelchair. Common causes of depression include despair, isolation, and labeling by others.

Despair

Immediately following my accident, I was concerned about all that I could no longer do. I had no experience with handicapped people, and my outlook was quite negative. I was focusing on all the problems. Even though the hospital staff brought me lots of magazines, videos, and literature on all the things that were possible, I wasn't ready to see myself in this new life. I found myself engaged in a lot of negative talk, saying things like, "I'll never be able to do that again!" It is easy to fall into a hole of self-pity, which can lead to depression.

What hit me next concerned my job. In this society, we are often led to measure our self-worth by the status of our job or how much we earn. I had most recently been a salesman, and the dollars I earned had been the measure of my success. Although it was possible for me to return to the same profession, I knew it would be significantly more difficult.

Sexuality can be a problem to deal with. With limited body function, it is easy to question what value we have to offer a partner. The change from the way sex used to be can be scary. Although persons with paralysis can have significantly fulfilling sexual experiences, they are different from traditional sexual activities. The strength of personal relationships is tested by a serious accident leading to paralysis. Some partners cannot deal with the situation, while others provide a wealth of love and support. The uncertainty of all this can add to depression.

Isolation

In the first few months after my accident, I received many cards, letters, and visits from friends and acquaintances while in the hospital. Upon returning home, the number of visits dropped off as people returned to their busy lives. My daily routine became significantly less active than before my accident. I found myself isolated and spending more time watching television and sleeping. In recent years, there has been great progress in efforts to make communities handicapped accessible. But as anyone in a wheelchair knows, there are many obstacles and barriers that prohibit us from freely going wherever we choose. It is easy to view the world as being full of steps, curbs, high counters, small hallways, hard-to-open doors, steep ramps, and bumps in the road. When one is feeling low, it is tempting to avoid these obstacles and stay home. This type of isolation can lead to depression.

Labeling

Labeling, the simple classification of a person by placing him or her into a category, can have a devastating effect on some people. Years ago, a person who was paralyzed was referred to as a cripple. This had a very negative connotation. So it became more acceptable to refer to paralyzed persons as handicapped. Then some people began to take offense to the word handicapped because it focuses on the disability, so a new phrase was coined—physically challenged. Some people take offense to the use of this term, saying it goes too far by attempting to sugar-coat the situation. I know people who prefer to be referred to as super-abled, since it takes more effort for them to accomplish a goal than it does for an able-bodied person. I never objected to being called a paraplegic, but I have friends that do. They see the use of the label "paraplegic" as demeaning. They prefer to be called a person with paraplegia, which focuses on the person, not the disability. Whatever the reason, if any kind of labeling bothers you, it adds to your frustration.

Avoiding Depression

Without a doubt, the influence of friends and loved ones makes a significant difference in how you feel. I have been blessed with a supporting family and encouraging people who inspire me, like Dr. Burdenko. When Christopher Reeve (the actor who played Superman) was hurt, his good friend Robin Williams came to the hospital to cheer him up. In order to be happy and involved in life, it certainly helps to surround yourself with friends. Unfortunately, not everyone is lucky enough to have such good friends.

To make friends, you need to take an active part in creating and maintaining relationships. I especially want to give this message to the families of those who are in a wheelchair. Make it a point to keep the person in the wheelchair socially active. A good place to start is with other wheelchair users who can share their experiences. There are many support and social groups for those in wheelchairs, especially sporting clubs.

As you recover from the trauma of your accident, become more active. Get out and exercise. Attend sporting and cultural events. Get involved with organizations and clubs. Meet and converse with other people in similar situations. Get out into the fresh air and exercise. Try new and different activities that you haven't tried before. Start to explore all the things that you can do. Put yourself into the frame of mind that you can do anything you want. You may have to do it differently from the way most people do it, but get out there and do it.

Instead of just plodding along each day, assess the situation and make a plan for what you want to do with your life. Set goals. You can be whatever you want to be. Surround yourself with people who can help you achieve your goals. The extent to which you can participate will be moderated by your abilities. Just take it slow at first and strive toward goals that are reasonable and achievable.

As my good friend Dr. Burdenko often says, "Work hard with a smile and exercise as much as you can for your mind and body. Never give up!"

Treating Depression

For many, depression following such a life-changing event as paralysis is inevitable. Depression may be so immediate and severe that there is no time to practice the above techniques for avoiding it. For these people, treatment is necessary.

Psychotherapy is a common and effective treatment for depression. Both individual and group therapy sessions are helpful. Some find the one-on-one intensive aspect of individual psychotherapy to be most helpful, while others prefer the emotional support of group psychotherapy. Cognitive therapy is often used to help change a person's negative thinking.

Many doctors use psychotherapy in conjunction with medication. There are many types of antidepressant medications, including selective serotonin reuptake inhibitors (SSRIs), tricyclics, and monoamine oxidase inhibitors. Talk to your doctor about which may be best for you. Many find that a combination of short-term medication and psychotherapy are extremely effective in helping people suffering with depression adjust to the changes in their lives.

There are also several natural treatments for depression. St. John's wort has been found to be a very effective herbal treatment for depression; in fact, it is as effective as most prescription drugs, without the side effects. Kava, another herbal remedy generally used in the treatment of anxiety, enhances the antidepressant effects of St. John's wort. A new supplement, S-adenosyl-L-methionine (SAM-e) is also effective as a treatment for depression. SAM-e is a substance produced naturally by the body. It is needed for the proper function of neurotransmitters in the brain.

You may or may not have to deal with pain in your daily life. If your pain is acute, it will diminish as your body heals. As you exercise, pay attention to what your body is telling you. Do not exercise when in pain. If your pain is chronic, do your best to divert your attention from it and keep from dwelling on the discomfort. Participate in activities that are mentally challenging, enjoyable, and intriguing.

Feeling sorrowful can be a problem for all types of people who are restricted to wheelchairs. So here are a few of my guidelines to avoid depression:

- Stay active with friends. Meet and socialize with people every day. Do not isolate yourself.

- Don't let yourself engage in negative thought. Instead of dwelling on all the things you can't do, focus on the activities that you can do.

- Improve your health through diet and exercise. You will feel better.

- Set goals you can achieve that will add value to your life. Then participate in activities to achieve these goals.

- Travel as much as you can to see new places and new faces.

Time is a great healer. As I look back, I remember that it was difficult for me cope with my new situation—both with the pain and the paraplegia. Now when I look at all the possibilities in my life, they seem limitless. To be sure, it is different from the way it was before, but nonetheless, there are plenty of opportunities. It took the passing of time to come to this realization.

SEVEN

Planning Your Program

Taking care of yourself with a program of health care and physical conditioning is extremely important during the rehabilitation phase. It is equally important for your continued well-being. You should plan this program as a lifestyle that you will follow for the rest of your life. This new lifestyle will include plenty of deep breathing exercises, proper nutrition, a positive frame of mind, and exercise on the land and in the water.

The sooner you begin living this lifestyle, the more you will benefit. The first thing to do is stop any bad habits that have a negative effect on your health, such as smoking, excessive drinking of alcohol, use of drugs, poor eating practices, and negative thinking. It may be difficult to make changes; however, the important thing is that you make a commitment to take care of yourself. Once you have made this commitment, you can start changing your habits. So the time to begin is now.

The next step is to give your body the supplies it needs to heal and stay healthy. This means an abundant supply of oxygen, nutritious foods, and plenty to drink.

Next, plan your exercises. The exercises will condition the muscles and reflexes that are already functional and stimulate those that need healing. Exercising in the water is an essential part of the Burdenko Method. The time you spend in the water, however, will be only a small part of your day. Even if you build up to a full hour in the water, most of your day will be spent on dry land. So exercising in the wheelchair is also an important part of your new lifestyle.

In this chapter, I will give you guidelines for planning your program for health and physical conditioning.

THE PREPARATORY PHASE

For a safe and effective exercise session, you must begin preparing long before the warm-up.

Get a Physical Checkup

Before starting any rehabilitation or conditioning program, you should get your doctor's permission. A physical checkup is needed to ensure that there are not any medical conditions present that will restrict your activity. Your doctor should weigh you and check your resting and post-exercise pulse, as well as the rest of your vital signs. Have your blood pressure tested. Retain the blood-pressure readings, and review this information from time to time as you have your blood pressure rechecked.

Attain the Proper Mindset

As mentioned in Chapter 2, the Burdenko Method emphasizes the stimulation of the nerves as integral to recovery from paralysis. Many of the exercises shown in this book illustrate body movements that do not appear possible for a person who is paralyzed. It is important to see how the body is supposed to function to attain a mindset in which you envision yourself fully capable of all movements. Use this mindset when performing the exercises to wake up and revitalize damaged or dysfunctional nerves.

In the early stages of the exercise program, you will focus on performing the exercises without paying too much attention to the paralyzed nerves. Then as you progress, the exercises will incorporate efforts to stimulate and move the paralyzed parts of your body. Here, your mindset will play an increasingly important role in helping the body heal itself. Many of the exercises include suggestions for developing the right mindset.

Set Realistic Goals

There are many different factors to consider when setting your goals, including your age, extent of injury, state of health, prior experience, and time available for training. We are each different. Some of us progress faster than others. Allow for ups and downs. I recall that when I began working with Dr. Burdenko, he told me that my rehabilitation would have waves. I would make progress, and then have some setbacks. The important thing was to keep at it, always moving in the right direction. This is especially true after an injury or if you have not exercised in a long time. Sometimes, you will fall back and not be able to accomplish the exercises you did a few weeks ago. This is a common occurrence in rehabilitation. Don't worry. That is just the way it works.

Make your goals obtainable. For example, if you are paraplegic, your first goal might be to perform twenty minutes of exercises in the water without becoming totally exhausted. Your next goal might be to balance while sitting on the water barbell for thirty seconds without the use of your hands. When you achieve your goals, set new ones of greater difficulty. In this manner, you will not feel overwhelmed by the whole program.

Select the Appropriate Exercises

The exercises in this book have been separated into two categories: land and water exercises. In each category, the exercises have been grouped according to the equipment used. Within each of these groups, I have listed the exercises in the order that I used in my reconditioning plan. What was difficult for me may be easy for you. So we recommend that you take some time to look over the exercises and select the ones that you feel are appropriate. And don't forget to consult with your doctor before starting.

Your workout should be a combination of land and water exercises. Always, always, always start with deep breathing exercises. Then select some easy land-based exercises for your warm-up. In the beginning, you may want to proceed from the warm-up directly to the water. When you are in better condition, you may want to add some land exercises after the warm-up, and then go to the water. On the days you do not work out in the water, be sure to do your land exercises.

Choose exercises that work the body in both directions. Some are well-suited for this, including walking in the water, arm circles, and neck rolls. These can be done both forward and backward. Other exercises use only one-half of a muscle pair. For example, push-ups in the wheelchair only work the muscles in the back of your upper arms (the triceps). An appropriate exercise to balance this muscle group would be arm curls with weights or exercise tubing. This uses the muscles in the front of your upper arms (the biceps).

Next, select exercises that are appropriate for your level of recovery and conditioning. In keeping with the Burdenko Method, your workouts should work on the following capabilities, progressing in the following order:

1. Balance.

2. Coordination.

3. Flexibility.

4. Endurance.

5. Speed.

6. Strength.

So the obvious question is: "What exercises should you use for each of the different capabilities?" The answer is that the same exercise may be used to develop each different capability. The important thing is the way in which the exercise is used. The intensity you use, the number of repetitions, the resistance you add, the distance you move, and the amount of concentration you can employ all play a part in determining the use for each exercise.

As you progress through the exercises, you will most likely notice a significant improvement in your physical capabilities. Exercises in the water are particularly useful for seeing results when parts of your body that have been paralyzed start to move. At first, there may be no movement at all. Then after some time, you may start to see small (micro) movements. Turn those micro movements into full functioning. It may take months, or it may take years. As the intensity of the exercises increase, move from dangling in the deep water to touching the bottom of the pool. Then go from touching the pool bottom in chest-deep water to actually standing. Gradually, move to shallower and shallower water. Eventually, you may be able to walk right out of the water and onto the land.

Select the Time and Place

Naturally, at first you need to ease into a program of daily exercise. Your body may be able to tolerate only short sessions, which is perfectly fine. The important thing is to set aside a time to exercise, and stick to it.

Whenever possible, exercise outdoors in fresh air and sunshine. A pleasant environment will positively affect your attitude. Being outside gives you a sense of freedom. After my accident, I moved from the suburbs of Boston to the beautiful mountains of northern New Hampshire. It is exhilarating to be outside in the country on a beautiful day in the fresh air. You can feel the difference!

A typical exercise session is a combination of land and water exercises, consisting of thirty minutes on the land, and thirty minutes in the water. The ideal situation would be to spend a part of each day in the water. You may be more comfortable starting with exercising two or three times a week, and eventually building up to exercising once a day. If you use an indoor pool, do your wheelchair warm-ups and deep breathing outdoors or away from any chlorine fumes in the air.

Wheelchair exercises do not offer the benefit of buoyancy that water provides, so exercises are more strenuous on land. Your wheelchair workouts should be planned accordingly. I prefer two short sessions—one in the morning and one in the evening. Try to select an outside location where you can enjoy the natural light, trees, birds, green grass, and fresh air.

It is important to change the location of your exercises frequently: try the bedroom, the living room, in front of a window, the back yard, the patio, the park, with family, with friends, etc. Exercise with music. Variety will keep it interesting!

THE EXERCISE SESSION

The workout program should be divided between land and water. Make deep-breathing exercises a priority at least twice a day. Dr. Burdenko and I usually incorporate deep breathing into our exercise sessions. However, if your daily schedule does not include at least two exercise sessions, set aside times for deep breathing. Begin exercising on the land and then proceed into the water. Whenever you exercise, your routine should consist of three distinct phases:

- The warm-up.
- The workout.
- The cool-down.

The Warm-Up

Begin each exercise session with a gentle warm-up routine. The warm-up consists of deep breathing, stretching, light exercises, and shaking. It should last about ten minutes. Warming up serves several purposes: It loosens the joints, limbers up the muscles and helps them relax, gets the blood pumping, and stimulates breathing. As the name implies, the warm-up is used to raise the temperature in the muscles. The increased temperature aids in metabolism and provides energy to the muscles. This makes for a more beneficial workout.

If the water temperature where you exercise is cooler than the air temperature, do your warm-up on land. This will get your system working efficiently before you enter the water. If you use an indoor pool, try to perform your warm-up outside in the fresh air.

This is also a good time to work on your frame of mind. Start thinking about what it will be like in the future when your body is better. Visualize the oxygen in your lungs going into the blood. Picture it traveling through the arteries. In your mind, see your nerves and muscles using the oxygen and nutrients in the blood to heal your body. Psyche yourself up!

The Workout

Always try to use a combination of land and water exercises for your workout. Change your routine frequently to keep it interesting. If you have to travel to a gym or health club to use a pool, you may find that you use this gym time to exercise primarily in the water. If so, set aside a different time to perform your land-based exercises.

If you are just beginning to use the water for exercise, you may find it much easier to move your body than you expected. You may even overexert yourself. Don't rush into a complete program of exercise. Use the water as a gentle tool, and gradually build up to a good aerobic workout.

Select appropriate exercises based on your level of rehabilitation, conditioning, and training. Remember to work in both directions. Select exercises that use both members of opposing muscle groups. For example, use the biceps to flex the arms. Then use the triceps to extend your arms. Over time, proceed from one level of exercise to the next in the proper order:

- Balance.
- Coordination.
- Flexibility.
- Endurance.
- Strength.
- Speed.

In the beginning, do the exercises slowly with body awareness to help avoid mistakes. If an exercise causes pain, stop and try a different one. As you start to increase your abilities, perform exercises in repetitions (reps). Start with a small number—one or two sets of ten repetitions—and take it nice and easy without reaching your pain threshold. Build up to three sets of ten repetitions. After thirty repetitions, set a new goal: ten slow repetitions, ten repetitions at a moderate speed, and ten fast repetitions. Our experience shows that this will improve your results. Remember to shake frequently, especially after a strenuous set of repetitions.

The Cool-Down

Cooling down is often overlooked, but it is just as important as warming up. This is where you gradually decrease your activity and let the body relax. Cooling down gently slows the pulse rate, reducing stress on the heart. Stretching the muscles helps them maintain flexibility after a workout. This will minimize soreness in the muscles and avoid stiffness in the joints.

Dr. Burdenko and I believe that muscles have a memory. If you are tired and do not take time to cool down, your muscles will remember the workout and feel sore all day. So it is very beneficial to perform your cool-down.

RELAXATION

Not only is it important to exercise to overcome paralysis, it is also important to rest, both physically and mentally, so that your body has a chance to recuperate. This section explains the importance of physical and mental relaxation.

Physical Relaxation

During rehabilitation, as you work your muscles, give them time to relax. Don't be in a hurry. After each exercise on the land, remember to shake. In the water, take time to float and give the muscles a rest before going on to the next exercise. You must also be sure to rest from exercise at least two days a week.

During later stages of conditioning, you may desire an aerobic workout where you increase the tempo and duration of your exercises. In this case, be sure to include a cool-down period to stretch and relax.

Mental Relaxation

Mental relaxation is actually a combination of physical relaxation and resting the mind in a peaceful state. This is a time to release stress. Relaxation is an event that you can plan during the day. When you relax, find a quiet environment and close your eyes. You should be in a contemplative state, almost like praying, deeply involved in meditation. You can relax in the water as well as on land. Some of Igor's students practice Yoga techniques and find that it helps them to relax as well.

THE PLAN

This program is designed for people with paraplegia; specifically, people who are paralyzed from the chest down but still have full use of their arms. When Dr. Burdenko and I started working together, the focus was on conditioning both the mind and body. The program progressed from simple to complex exercises. The main emphasis was on developing those abilities I had lost since my injury. The number of exercises at each session depended upon my condition. On some days, I could do many exercises, and other days I could not tolerate any. We adjusted each session accordingly—never pushing me beyond my limit.

In each exercise, we focused on a particular ability: balance, flexibility, coordination, endurance, strength, and speed. As time progressed, Dr. Burdenko made the exercises more fun and challenging, always emphasizing body awareness and making sure that I performed the exercises correctly without any kind of adaptation. I saw him once a week. During the rest of the week, I practiced on my own—sometimes a few days a week, sometimes more. I kept track of the exercises in a notebook for my future reference.

After a few months, Dr. Burdenko emphasized the importance of my mindset while exercising. He had me concentrate on waking up the nerves and muscles that had been paralyzed. More and more, I tried to use my legs in the water, always straining to regain their use. This should become a basic part of your program as well.

In this book, we do not recommend a certain number of repetitions for each exercise, because everyone is different. What was easy for me may be difficult for you. Always exercise without pain. If an exercise causes pain, then stop and try a different one. Start with a small number of repetitions and slowly increase to thirty. Then work on the exercises at different speeds: slow, moderate, and fast.

You should start with a realistic review of your current health and physical condition. My situation looked like this:

- Paraplegic—unable to move anything below the chest.

- Chronic pain in the upper body and right arm.

- Normal blood pressure.

- Overweight with poor eating habits.

- Reduced breathing volume; unable to cough or sneeze.

- Lacking balance and the ability to stay upright when leaning forward or to the sides.

- Relatively good range of motion from daily stretching.

- Weak muscles in the upper body, making it difficult to transfer into and out of the wheelchair.

- Limited endurance; difficulty in propelling the wheelchair over a distance or up an incline.

Based on this information, Dr. Burdenko and I created the following exercise schedule for me, which I still follow today:

I start off each day early in the morning with stretching and deep breathing.

In the midmorning, when I have the most energy of the day, I do the bulk of my exercises five days of the week. I either go into the water or do a land workout session. My water workout always begins with a warm-up period on the land. After I have stretched and done some deep breathing and a few light exercises, I proceed into the water. I end my workout, slowing the pace of my exercises and doing my cool-down in the water. If the water temperature is chilly, I relax in the Jacuzzi for about three minutes.

In the afternoon, I do my mind conditioning with visualization and meditation for about twenty minutes.

In the evening, I do a light session of land exercises five days a week.

The ideal situation for me is to exercise on land for twenty to thirty minutes twice a day. I try to exercise in the water for about forty-five minutes at least five times a week. In actuality, I have to govern my activity by the amount of pain I have. Sometimes I have to cut my sessions short. On some days, I cannot tolerate any exercise.

The following table shows the order in which I progressed through the exercises.

LAND-BASED PROGRAM

Week	Land Exercise #	Total Workout Time	Frequency
1 & 2	1,2,3,4,5,6	10 min.	Once a day, 3 times a week.
3	7,8	10 min.	Once a day, 3 times a week.
4	9	10 min.	Once a day, 3 times a week.
5	10,11,12	10 min.	Once a day, 5 times a week.
6	15	10 min.	Once a day, 5 times a week.
7	13,14	10 min.	Once a day, 5 times a week.
8	15,16,43,44	10 min.	Once a day, 5 times a week.
9	Same as above	10 min.	Once a day, 3 times a week; and on alternate days, twice a day, 2 times a week.
10	17,18,19,20	10 min.	Once a day, 3 times a week; and on alternate days, twice a day, 2 times a week.
11 & 12	45,46	10 min.	Once a day, 3 times a week; and on alternate days, twice a day, 2 times a week.
13	21,22,23	20 min.	Once a day, 2 times a week; and on alternate days, twice a day, 3 times a week.
14	47,48	20 min.	Once a day, 2 times a week; and on alternate days, twice a day, 3 times a week.
15	24,25	20 min.	Once a day, 2 times a week; and on alternate days, twice a day, 3 times a week.
16	30	20 min.	Once a day, 2 times a week; and on alternate days, twice a day, 3 times a week.
17	26,27,28,29	20 min.	Once a day, 2 times a week; and on alternate days, twice a day, 3 times a week.
18	30,31,32	20 min.	Once a day, 2 times a week; and on alternate days, twice a day, 3 times a week.
19	39,40,41	20 min.	Once a day, 2 times a week; and on alternate days, twice a day, 3 times a week.

Week	Land Exercise #	Total Workout Time	Frequency
20	33,34,42	20 min.	Twice a day, 5 times a week.
21	49,50	20 min.	Once a day, 2 times a week; and on alternate days, twice a day, 3 times a week.
22	35,36	20 min.	Once a day, 2 times a week; and on alternate days, twice a day, 3 times a week.
23	37,38,51,52	20 min.	Once a day, 2 times a week; and on alternate days, twice a day, 3 times a week.
24	53,54	20 min.	Once a day, 2 times a week; and on alternate days, twice a day, 3 times a week.

WATER-BASED PROGRAM

Week	Water Exercise #	Total Workout Time	Frequency
1	1,2,3,4,5	20 min.	Once a day, 3 times a week.
2 & 3	6,7,8,9	20 min.	Once a day, 3 times a week.
4	10,11,12	20 min.	Once a day, 3 times a week.
5	36,37	20 min.	Once a day, 5 times a week.
6 & 7	13,14,15	20 min.	Once a day, 5 times a week.
8	28,29,30,31	20 min.	Once a day, 5 times a week.
9	35, 16, 17, 18	30 min.	Once a day, 3 times a week; and on alternate days, twice a day, twice a week.
10	33, 53, 55	30 min.	Once a day, 3 times a week; and on alternate days, twice a day, twice a week.
11	19, 55	30 min.	Once a day, 3 times a week; and on alternate days, twice a day, twice a week.
12	38, 39	30 min.	Once a day, 3 times a week; and on alternate days, twice a day, twice a week.
13	20, 59, 60	30 min.	Once a day, twice a week; and on alternate days, twice a day, 3 times a week.

Week	Water Exercise #	Total Workout Time	Frequency
14 & 15	40, 41 42 ,43, 44	30 min.	Once a day, twice a week; and on alternate days, twice a day, 3 times a week.
16	45, 46	30 min.	Once a day, twice a week; and on alternate days, twice a day, 3 times a week.
17	21, 32, 34	30 min.	Once a day, twice a week; and on alternate days, twice a day, 3 times a week.
18	47, 48, 49	30 min.	Once a day, twice a week; and on alternate days, twice a day, 3 times a week.
19	22, 23, 56, 57	30 min.	Once a day, twice a week; and on alternate days, twice a day, 3 times a week.
20	50, 51	30 min.	Twice a day, 5 times a week.
21	24, 25, 60	45 min.	Twice a day, 5 times a week.
22	52	45 min.	Twice a day, 5 times a week.
23	26, 27	45 min.	Twice a day, 5 times a week.
24	58	45 min.	Twice a day, 5 times a week.

Each week, you will add new exercises to your routine. As you progress in your exercises, you will advance from exercises that are relatively easy to ones that are more challenging. Your total workout time should be about an hour. In order to keep your workout time within this period, you will have to minimize and eliminate some of the exercises from previous weeks. As I add exercises from week to week, I select those previous exercises that I found most beneficial and alternate through those day to day. Work with your physical therapist to decide which exercises you need to keep as part of your routine and which you can eliminate based upon how helpful they are for you and how well you are able to perform them.

The only person who can select the best plan for you to be healthy and physically fit and to recover from paralysis is you. To be sure, you need to seek the advice of professionals (doctors and physical therapists), but the formulation of a plan and the motivation to carry out that plan is up to you. The Burdenko Method relies on exercises on the land and in the water to change your body performance and promote the healing process.

Your exercise plan should include a routine for when, where, and how you exercise during the day. Each exercise session should include a warm-up, workout, and cool-down phase. The exercises should progress to improve the following abilities in this order: balance, coordination, flexibility, endurance, strength, and speed. To stimulate nerve regeneration, you should have a mindset in which you visualize the nerves working and attempt to move the paralyzed parts of your body.

Exercises in the water are best for seeing the results when the paralyzed parts of your body start to move. At first, you will exercise where the water is deep, letting the water support you. As function returns to your body, move from deep water to shallow water, and begin using your legs to support your weight.

As the power of movement returns to your legs, you will notice only micromovements at first. Then as you continue to perform the exercises while visualizing in your mind your legs moving fully, you may find that your paralysis is going away and that you are regaining the use of your legs. At first, the muscles will be weak, and it will be challenging to use your legs. As you exercise in the water, concentrate on stretching your legs out straight and touching the bottom of the pool. As you gain more and more control of your legs, gradually move into the shallow water and try to stand on the bottom. First do this in shallow water and continue your progression until you are able to walk out of the pool.

If at all possible, you should do at least part of your water workout in salt water where you will be more buoyant. This will make your water workouts a little easier. If you are able to exercise in the ocean in a cove where the water is smooth, you can transition from exercising in deep water to shallower water, and slowly work your way up onto the beach. This may take several weeks or several months depending upon your level of injury and the amount of effort you put into your recovery. Walking on land will at first require additional support in the form of crutches or braces in the beginning. The goal is to walk freely without support and regain full use of your body.

I intend to walk right up the steps and out of the pool one day. I used to think it was impossible, but now I know that it can be done. All I need is a plan to get there, and the mindset to make it happen.

Geoffrey Allanbrook's Story

I broke my neck in a diving accident in June of 1994. I was quadriplegic and knew only of traditional methods of physical therapy, which gave me little to look forward to. My expectations were changed dramatically when I recently learned about Dr. Burdenko from a friend of mine, who also was quadriplegic. After working with Dr. Burdenko, he now walks with braces and crutches.

Dr. Burdenko's holistic approach gives advantages that traditional Western medicine cannot. He never sets limits on what his clients can do. Since working with Igor over the past few months, I have been able to move my legs in the water. I stood waist-deep in the water on my own, and I took my first steps in the water. I feel certain that in the coming months, I will be able to walk on land.

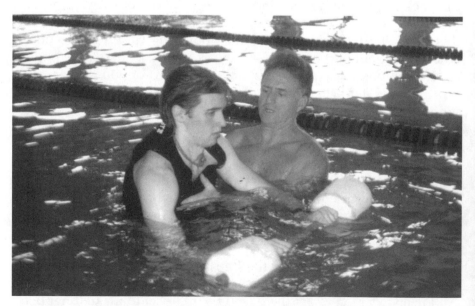

Geoffrey Allanbrook working out in the water with Dr. Burdenko.

PART TWO

Land
Exercises

EIGHT

Land Exercise Basics

This part of the book deals with exercises on the land—more specifically, exercises done in the wheelchair. They are ideally suited for a program to help recover from paraplegia; however, the exercises could be useful to anyone in a wheelchair. Most of the exercises involve movement of the upper body, which may be of benefit to most people who are wheelchair-bound due to polio, stroke, injury, amputation, or a variety of other conditions.

This section begins with some general guidelines about wheelchair exercising and the equipment you can use, followed by the exercises. The exercises are grouped according to the equipment used and are not necessarily in order of difficulty. Exercises with no equipment are listed first. If you desire to work your way through the exercises in a logical progression, refer to the exercise plan in Chapter 7.

SAFETY ISSUES

Check with your doctor, physical therapist, or health-care practitioner before starting a physical-therapy program. You should make sure that there are no health problems that may prevent you from exercising or following any of the recommendations in this book.

Here are a few safety guidelines to follow when exercising in a wheelchair:

- Locate your wheelchair on level ground and lock the brakes.

- Make sure there is adequate clearance allowing you to swing your arms and bend in any direction without obstructions.

- When attempting new exercises that involve bending and leaning, have an assistant with you in case you need help.

- Do not hold your breath while exercising.

- Do not exercise immediately after a meal.

- Do not continue a particular exercise if it causes pain.

- Check your blood pressure from time to time to make sure you are not placing too much stress on your heart.

EQUIPMENT

Most of the exercises in the wheelchair can be performed without any special equipment. The same exercises can be increased in difficulty by adding simple stretchable tubing and light weights for resistance.

Exercise Tubing

Tubing provides resistance when stretched, taking the place of a bulky set of weights. The exercise tubing is used both in the water and on the land. I use common surgical tubing obtainable at most medical supply stores and some drugstores. The inside of the tubing is five-sixteenths of an inch in diameter, and the tubing is made from natural latex rubber that is one-sixteenth of an inch thick.

To get started, you will need two 2-foot-long pieces and two 13-foot-long pieces (including the loops). You should tie a loop at the end of each piece of tubing large enough for your hand or foot to fit through. (See Figure 8.1.) The loop also provides a means of attaching to the wheelchair by wrapping around the frame and passing the

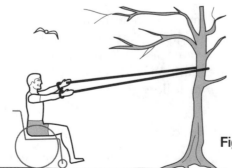

Figure 8.1. Exercising with tubing.

other end back through the loop. The advantage of using tubing instead of flat elastic bands is that it is easy to tie and untie.

Tubing will wear out with use. Always inspect the tubing and replace it when it has cracks or shows any sign of wear.

Water Barbells

Water barbells are made from a plastic tube with floats at each end. (See Figure 8.2.) Although these barbells are designed primarily to be used in the water, they are useful for adding a minimum amount of resistance when used on the land. The light weight of these items makes them ideal for holding with arms extended for exercises that work on improving upper-body balance. They provide a good transition from exercising with no equipment to exercising with wrist weights.

Weights

Wrist weights (sometimes called ankle weights) can be used to increase the difficulty of wheelchair exercises. These are padded weights that wrap around your wrists or ankles and attach with a Velcro strap. (See Figure 8.3.) The weights come in different hefts, usually 1, $2^1/_2$, 5, $7^1/_2$, and 10 pounds. The set I use is adjustable. It has individual pockets that hold weights in half-pound increments.

As your strength improves, wrist weights can be added for just about any of the wheelchair exercises in this book; however, a word of caution is advisable. The added weight may throw you off balance when you least expect it. When attached to your wrist, the weight will affect your balance as you extend your arm away from your centerline. You may have the arm strength to lift the weight, but you may not have the abdominal or back muscles to maintain your stability.

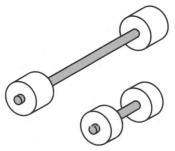

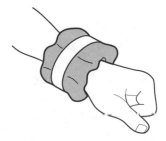

Figure 8.2. Water barbells.   **Figure 8.3.** Wrist weights.

WHEELCHAIR POSTURE

I group wheelchairs into three basic styles, each affecting the way you sit. First is the all-purpose traditional style that has been around for years. This has a straight back and level seat. It may or may not be motorized. The next type of wheelchair has been designed for a more active lifestyle. This is the style that I use. It is lighter in weight, and the seat is tilted back slightly. The third type is designed specifically for sports, like basketball, tennis, etc. The seat in this chair has been tilted back at a much greater angle to accommodate leaning and bending motions.

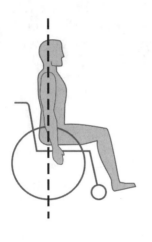

Figure 8.4.
Proper wheelchair posture.

Sit erect whenever you exercise in a wheelchair. (See Figure 8.4.) Your spine should be long and straight (maintaining its natural curve) all the way up from your pelvis to the top of your head. Your neck should be long with your head lifted, looking straight forward. Shoulders should be pressed back and down but relaxed. This position lifts the chest for deep breathing.

If the seat back of your chair is angled, you may find it helpful to use a lumbar support, or a small cushion behind your lower back. A rolled-up towel will work just fine. In the future, we hope you will not need this support.

INCREASING THE LEVEL OF DIFFICULTY
OF YOUR EXERCISES

As you become proficient in the exercises, you may desire to make them more challenging. The first step is to increase the number of repetitions. The next step is to perform the repetitions at different speeds: slow, medium, and fast.

Another way to make the exercises more difficult is to add resistance. Some of the land exercises can be performed with a small water barbell held in each hand. This will add a very small amount of weight. Just about all of the land-based exercises can be performed with wrist weights. The advantage of wrist weights is they wrap around each wrist, leaving your hands free. Start off by adding a very small amount of weight—one-half or one pound—equally to each wrist. The weights will affect your balance, so be cautious each time you add weight. Gradually add more weight, up to about 5 pounds.

Exercise in Both Directions

Most exercises with tubing can be performed in the reverse direction. For exercises in which tubing is attached to a pole in front, you can turn the chair around. The same exercise can then be performed with the tubing anchored from behind.

Similarly, the motion of the arms can be done in reverse. For example, if you are circling in a forward direction, you can vary the exercise by circling your arms in a backward direction. Be creative, and try to exercise all the muscles in your body.

Exercise With Tubing

Exercise tubing provides resistance when stretched. The amount of resistance can be varied by: doubling the tubing, removing the slack between you and the anchor point, or varying the length of the tube. When you double the tubing, you must exert more force to pull it, since you are doubling the resistance. When there is slack in the length of the tubing, it lowers resistance, since little or no force is required to pull it. When you remove any remaining slack in the tubing, you increase the resistance. Adding length to your tubing decreases resistance, as less force is required to pull a longer tube, since a smaller percentage of the tubing is being stretched. As your strength improves, you may want to shorten the pieces to add more resistance.

You will need several different lengths of exercise tubing. The length of the tubing should be adjusted for each exercise so that in the relaxed position, there is just a slight amount of tension. In most cases, you can move the wheelchair closer or farther from the anchor point to remove any slack.

Exercises 43 through 46 use tubing secured to the wheelchair. Attach the tubing to the frame or to one of the spacers (the metal tubes that connect the hand wheel and the tire). This can be done simply by wrapping the tubing around the frame and threading it back through the loop at the end of the tubing. (See Figure 8.5 on page 90.) For some exercises (like the Triceps Extension and Arm Press), you may prefer to loop the tubing around the handles at the back of your wheelchair.

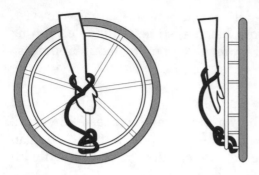

Figure 8.5. Securing tubing to the wheelchair.

Exercises 47 through 50 require a long piece of tubing attached to each hand and wrapped around a fixed object, such as a pole or doorknob, in front or behind you. This piece should be about 12 feet long. (See Figure 8.6, below.) Exercises 51 through 54 require two pieces of tubing. Each should be about 6 feet long. They will stretch out to the sides.

For exercises in which the tubing is tied together in a circle, simply hold the tubing in the palm of your hand with your thumb on the outside.

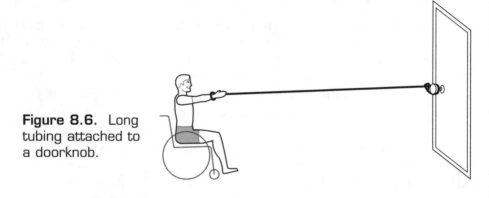

Figure 8.6. Long tubing attached to a doorknob.

For exercises that use long pieces of tubing, tie loops at each end. The loop should be just large enough for your hand to fit through and fit snugly around your wrist. (See Figure 8.7, below.) Looping the tubing around your wrist will prevent you from losing it if it slips out of your hand. Also, if you wrap it too tightly around the wrist, the circulation in your hand may be cut off. You may find it helpful to wear wheelchair gloves.

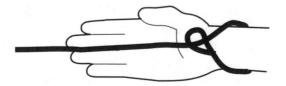

Figure 8.7. Looping tubing around hand.

ON TO THE EXERCISES

You are now ready to proceed to the exercises. Don't forget to begin each exercise session with deep-breathing exercises and a warm-up period. Relax and shake (see Chapter 5) between exercises, and include a cool-down period at the end. It is a good idea to exercise with a physical therapist or a friend to monitor your progress and physical condition. Do not exercise if you feel pain.

Work hard, with a smile, and exercise as much as you can for your mind and body.

Land Exercises

BASIC EXERCISES

1. Arm Swings Out
2. Picking Apples
3. Push Downs
4. Shoulder Shrugs
5. Pushups
6. Neck Rolls
7. Arm Stretch Forward
8. Arm Swings Up
9. Diagonal Twist
10. Count to Eight
11. Boxing in Front
12. Boxing to the Sides
13. Body Stretch Forward
14. Stretch Around the World
15. Arm Extensions to the Side
16. Shoulder Raises
17. Arm Swings Behind the Head
18. Palms Together
19. 5-Count Arm Raises
20. Arm Extensions
21. Stomach Roll
22. Tight Butt
23. Hip Moves
24. Reach Downs
25. Lower-Arm Raises
26. Diagonal Arm Circles
27. Arm Cranks
28. Arm Circles in Front
29. Arm Flutters
30. Twists
31. Push and Pull
32. Cross-Country Skiing
33. Lean Forward
34. Downhill Skiing
35. Clap Behind
36. Knee Pick-ups
37. Leg Kicks
38. Knee Lifts

BARBELL EXERCISES

39. Arm Circles With Barbells
40. Barbell Grab
41. Barbell Twists
42. Barbell Lift

TUBING EXERCISES

43. Curls
44. Triceps Extension
45. Arm Raise
46. Arm Circles to the Sides
47. Flying
48. Arm Circles With Tubing

49. Skiing
50. Arm Stretch With Tubing
51. Pull Downs
52. Cross Your Chest
53. Hug Yourself
54. Breaststroke

Land Exercise 1.
Arm Swings Out

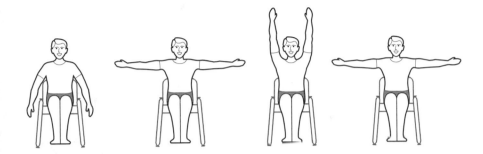

PURPOSE

This exercise serves as a wake-up call for the breathing center and improves balance. It stretches arm and shoulder muscles and increases range of motion (ROM) of shoulders and arms.

STARTING POSITION

Sit erect with arms down at sides.

ACTION

1. Swing arms straight out to sides at shoulder height. Inhale. Pause briefly.

2. Swing arms up straight over head. Exhale. Pause briefly.

3. Swing arms out straight to sides. Inhale. Pause briefly.

4. Return to starting position. Exhale.

COMMENTS

Maintain body awareness throughout the exercise. In the beginning, the upper body may sway as you raise the arms. Concentrate on maintaining balance and breathing deeply. Inhale through your nose and raise your chest, filling your lungs with air. As you exhale, purse your lips together and blow—like you would blow out a candle.

Land Exercise 2.
Picking Apples

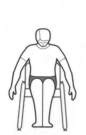 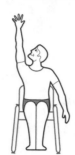 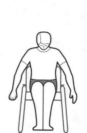 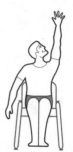

PURPOSE

This exercise increases the ROM of the neck, shoulders, upper arms, wrists, and hands, and improves deep breathing. It also stretches side (lateral), shoulder, and arm muscles.

STARTING POSITION

Sit erect with your arms down at your sides. Tilt your head down. Exhale.

ACTION

1. Bending your elbow, raise your right arm, keeping it alongside the body. Raise your arm straight over your head and stretch, spreading your fingers wide. Tilt your head up, and watch your hand. Inhale. Hold this position for 3 to 5 seconds.

2. Bring your arm straight down. Close your hand. Tilt your head down. Exhale.

3. Do the same with your left arm.

COMMENTS

Pretend you are picking apples from trees. Open your hand and stretch to reach up high. When you bing your arm down, close your hand. Concentrate on deep breathing. Expand your chest as you inhale. Purse your lips and blow all the air out as you bring your arms down.

Land Exercise 3.
Push Downs

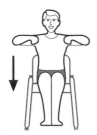 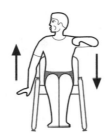 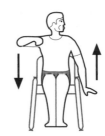

PURPOSE

This exercise improves balance, coordination, and ROM in the neck, shoulders, and arms.

STARTING POSITION

Sit erect with your arms held out at the sides at shoulder level and your elbows bent. Keep your hands clenched in fists with your palms down.

ACTION

1. Spread your right hand open and push your right arm straight down. Turn your head to the right.

2. Raise your right hand up to the starting position, clenching your fist. At the same time, open your left hand and push your left arm straight down. Turn your head left. Hold this position for two to three seconds.

COMMENTS

Focus on performing this exercise precisely. As you move your arms up and down, keep your hands flat (parallel to the floor). Raise and lower them vertically in straight lines. Maintain your upper-body balance. Pay attention to your breathing and coordination.

VARIATION

As your balance and coordination improve, add the following isometric exercise: Tighten and hold your arm muscles firm when your arm is raised up or pushed down.

Land Exercise 4.
Shoulder Shrugs

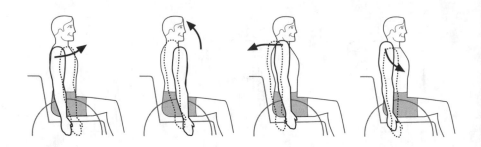

PURPOSE

This exercise increases ROM in the shoulders, reduces tension in the upper body, lifts your rib cage, and increases deep breathing.

STARTING POSITION

Sit erect with your arms down at your sides.

ACTION

1. Rotate your shoulders forward in a circle. Stretch them upward, bring them forward, and roll them down and back.

2. Now circle your shoulders in reverse, rotating the shoulders backward.

COMMENTS

Maintain body awareness. Stay erect, and only move the shoulders. Keep your arms relaxed and hanging down limp at the sides.

VARIATION

Perform this exercise at three different speeds: slow, medium, and fast.

Land Exercise 5.
Pushups

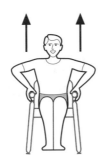 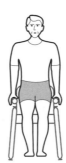

PURPOSE

This exercise strengthens the arms and lifts the body.

STARTING POSITION

Sit erect. Grasp the armrests of the wheelchair with each hand. If you have no armrests, grip the top of the tires. Inhale.

ACTION

1. Extend your arms, pushing your body up off the seat. Exhale.

2. Lower your body until your bottom is just above (but not touching) the seat. Inhale.

COMMENTS

Focus on fully extending both arms at the same time. Keep your elbows in close to the body. As your strength improves, perform sets of repetitions at different speeds: slow, moderate speed, and fast.

VARIATION

Each time you push up, turn your head in a different direction: left, right, up, down, straight ahead.

Land Exercise 6.
Neck Rolls

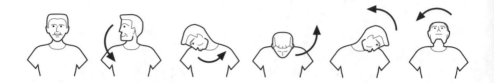

PURPOSE

This exercise increases the ROM of the neck and improves deep breathing.

STARTING POSITION

Sit erect with your arms down at your sides.

ACTION

1. Inhale, taking a deep breath. Look straight ahead.

2. Exhale and turn your head all the way to the right.

3. As you inhale, roll your head down and circle your neck to the left all the way around, bringing your head back up.

4. Looking straight ahead, exhale.

5. Perform the same actions in the opposite direction.

COMMENTS

This exercise helps coordinate neck motions with breathing.

VARIATION

Instead of rolling the head down in front, roll the head back.

Land Exercise 7.
Arm Stretch Forward

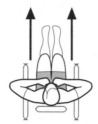 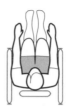

PURPOSE

This exercise improves upper-body balance and ROM in shoulders. It also develops strength in the upper arms and stretches the muscles in the hands.

STARTING POSITION

Sit erect with your arms out to the sides at shoulder level with your elbows bent and your hands clenched in front of your chest, with your palms facing downward.

ACTION

1. Extend both arms straight out in front. Open your hands and spread your fingers apart.

2. Bring your arms back in to the starting position. Clench your hands into a fist.

COMMENTS

This exercise will throw you off balance, and you may tip forward. If you cannot maintain your balance, only partially extend your arms.

As your balance improves, flex your arm muscles, making this an isometric exercise to build strength.

Land Exercise 8.
Arm Swings Up

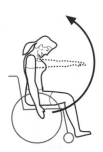 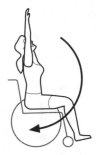 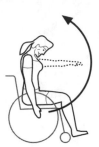 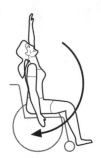

PURPOSE

This exercise stretches your neck, shoulder, and arm muscles.

STARTING POSITION

Sit erect with your arms down at your sides and your head lowered.

ACTION

1. Swing your right arm straight out in front and then up over your head in one continuous motion. Follow the motion of your arm with your head, looking straight up. Inhale. Hold this position for a moment.

2. Swing your arm back down. Again, follow the motion of your arm with your head. Exhale.

3. Perform the same actions with your left arm, moving your head as you go.

COMMENTS

In the beginning, it may be difficult to maintain your balance. Start by holding onto the tire of the wheelchair with one hand while raising the other arm. As strength and balance improve, let go of the wheel and let your arm hang down at your side. Concentrate on breathing deeply.

Land Exercise 9.
Diagonal Twist

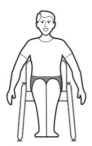 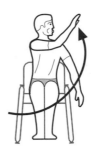

PURPOSE

This exercise improves upper-body balance. It also stretches the side (lateral), shoulder, and arm muscles and increases the ROM of shoulders and arms.

STARTING POSITION

Sit erect with your arms down at your sides.

ACTION

1. Turn your head and twist your upper body to the left. At the same time, extend and swing your right arm out diagonally over your left shoulder.

2. Return to the starting position.

3. Repeat this action, twisting to the right this time.

COMMENTS

The movement of your arm should be continuous. After your arm swings over the opposite shoulder, let it return to its starting position.

Land Exercise 10.
Count to Eight

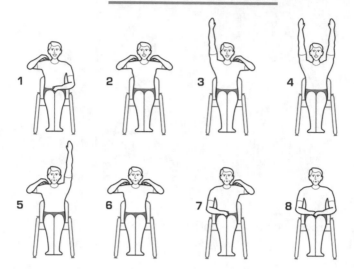

PURPOSE

This exercise improves upper-body balance. It also stretches the arm and shoulder muscles, increases ROM of shoulders and arms, and improves coordination.

STARTING POSITION

Sit erect with your hands in your lap.

ACTION

1. Raise your right arm, and with your elbow out to the side, put your right hand on your right shoulder.

2. With your right arm still on your right shoulder, raise your left arm, and with your elbow out to the side, put your left hand on your left shoulder.

3. Raise your right arm up straight over your head.

4. Raise your left arm up straight over your head.

5. Lower your right arm, and with your elbow out to the side, put your right hand on your right shoulder.

6. Lower your left arm, and with your elbow out to the side, put your left hand on your left shoulder.

7. Lower your right arm, and place your right hand in your lap.

8. Lower your left arm, and place your left hand in your lap.

COMMENTS

Count out each step to yourself. In the beginning, your body may wobble as you move your arms. Use the muscles in your back to maintain your balance. Fix your eyes on a spot on the wall in front of you to help maintain your balance.

VARIATION

Place your hands behind your head, instead of on your shoulders. Feel the stretch in your back muscles.

Land Exercise 11.
Boxing in Front

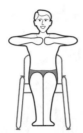 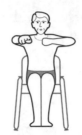 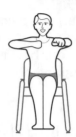

PURPOSE

This exercise improves upper-body balance. It also stretches the arm and shoulder muscles, increases ROM of your arms and wrists, and helps you concentrate on breathing.

STARTING POSITION

Sit erect with your arms up and your elbows bent outward at the same level as your shoulders, with your hands clenched in fists. Inhale.

ACTION

1. Punch your right arm out in front of you, turning your fist a bit to the left. Exhale.
2. Bring your right arm back into the chest, and at the same time, punch your left arm out. Inhale.
3. Continue boxing, alternating arm movements.

COMMENTS

Initially, you may have difficulty maintaining your balance. Concentrate on staying erect. Make moves slowly and correctly. When you can do this without wobbling, increase your speed. Keep your elbows at shoulder level. This position lifts the diaphragm, making it easier to breathe.

VARIATION

Use different style punches: jabs, uppercuts, etc.

Land Exercise 12.
Boxing to the Sides

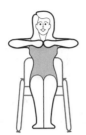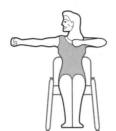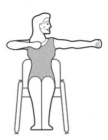

PURPOSE

This exercise improves upper-body balance; stretches your side, shoulder, and arm muscles; increases the ROM of your neck, arms, and wrists; and helps you concentrate on your breathing.

STARTING POSITION

Sit erect with your arms up and your elbows out to the sides at the same level as your shoulders. Make fists with your hands. Inhale.

ACTION

1. Punch your right arm out to the side while turning your head to the right. Exhale.
2. Return to the starting position. Inhale.
3. Repeat action on the left side.

COMMENTS

This exercise should be attempted after you master "Boxing in Front." Maintain body awareness throughout the exercise—maintain your balance and remain erect. Perform the exercise slowly at first, and then build up to a swift workout.

VARIATION

Combine "Boxing in Front" (page 102) with "Boxing to the Sides," punching alternately in front and to the side.

Land Exercise 13.
Body Stretch Forward

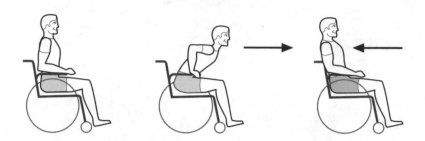

PURPOSE

This exercise improves balance and stretches and strengthens the upper-body muscles.

STARTING POSITION

Sit erect and hold onto the armrests of your wheelchair (or the top of the tires if you have no armrests). Inhale.

ACTION

1. Lean forward and stretch. Look straight ahead (keep your chin up). Exhale.

2. Lean back, returning to the starting position. Inhale.

MINDSET

Imagine that you are leaning, using only the abdominal and back muscles. Reteach those muscles to work. Coordinate in your mind the motion of your body with the movements those muscles would be making. Stimulate the nerves through visualization to help the body heal itself.

COMMENTS

Pay attention to your breathing. In the beginning, leaning will be controlled by the arms and possibly the back muscles. As strength improves, use your abdominal muscles more than your back muscles.

Land Exercise 14.
Stretch Around the World

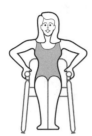 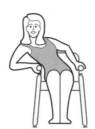 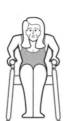 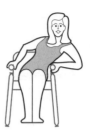

PURPOSE

This exercise improves balance and strengthens the side (lateral), back, and front muscles.

STARTING POSITION

Sit erect and hold onto the armrests (or tires if you have no armrests). Inhale.

ACTION

1. Lean your body to the right. Look straight ahead (chin up). Exhale halfway.

2. Lean forward. Look straight ahead (chin up). Exhale fully.

3. Lean left. Look straight ahead (chin up). Inhale halfway.

4. Lean back. Look straight ahead (chin up). Inhale all the way.

COMMENTS

In the beginning, your movement will be controlled by your arms. As you build up strength, use your upper-body muscles to move. As your flexibility improves, increase the distance that you stretch.

VARIATION

Perform sets of repetitions at different speeds. At slow speed, hold the stretch for a short time. Adjust your breathing accordingly.

Land Exercise 15.
Arm Extensions to the Side

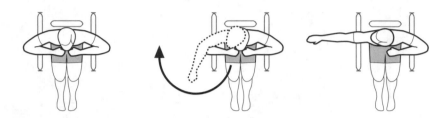

PURPOSE

This exercise increases ROM of the neck and shoulders and develops flexibility in the arms.

STARTING POSITION

Sit erect with your arms up at shoulder level, your elbows out to the sides, and your hands closed in front of your chest.

ACTION

1. Slowly swing your right arm forward, then out to the side, while opening your hand. Meanwhile, turn your head to the right, following the motion of your arm. Inhale.

2. Slowly bring your arm back in, closing your fist. Look straight ahead. Exhale.

3. Repeat this action with your left arm.

COMMENTS

Swinging your arm out in front may throw you off balance. If so, keep your arm closer to your body as you swing it out. Maintain proper body awareness. Concentrate on keeping your back straight. Keep your arm straight and level. Keep your elbows at shoulder height to raise your chest and increase your deep breathing. Coordinate the movement of your head with your arms.

Land Exercise 16.
Shoulder Raises

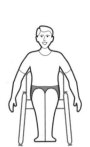 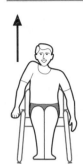 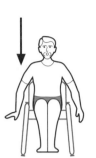 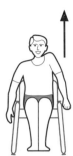

PURPOSE

This exercise helps you concentrate on body awareness, improves ROM in your shoulders, and stretches the side muscles.

STARTING POSITION

Sit erect with your arms down at your sides.

ACTION

1. Raise your right shoulder straight up. Close your right hand.

2. Relax your shoulder muscles, and drop your shoulder. Open your hand.

3. Perform the same actions with the other shoulder.

COMMENTS

Concentrate on body awareness. Sit up straight; don't bend forward. When raising your shoulder, use only the shoulder muscles; do not move your elbow. Let your arm hang down loose. When dropping your shoulder, relax your muscles and drop your arm quickly like a dead weight.

VARIATION

As an advanced exercise, move your neck up and down as your shoulder moves.

Land Exercise 17.
Arm Swings Behind the Head

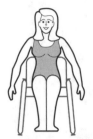 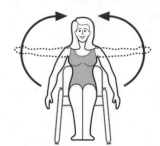 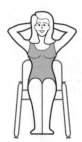

PURPOSE

This exercise improves upper-body balance and ROM in your shoulders. It also helps you maintain body awareness and improve your coordination.

STARTING POSITION

Sit erect with your arms down at your sides.

ACTION

1. Swing your arms straight out to your sides, then bend your elbows and place your hands behind your head. Inhale.

2. Return to the starting position. Exhale.

COMMENTS

Maintain body awareness while doing this exercise. Move your arms slowly and coordinate movements of each arm so that they move simultaneously. Keep your back straight. Initially, it may be difficult to maintain your balance. Locate a spot directly in front of you in the distance. Concentrate on the spot to help maintain balance.

VARIATION

Swing one arm at a time. This adds difficulty to balancing.

Land Exercise 18.
Palms Together

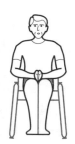 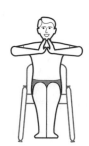 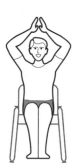

PURPOSE

This exercise improves upper-body balance and increases ROM in your shoulders, elbows, and wrists.

STARTING POSITION

Sit erect with the palms of your hands pressed together in front of your stomach, with your fingers pointing up (as if you were praying).

ACTION

1. Raise your arms to shoulder level with your palms together.

2. Raise your arms over your head with your palms together.

3. Lower your arms to shoulder level with your palms together.

4. Return to starting position.

COMMENTS

Concentrate on the position of your hands. Maintain even pressure on the hands. For an advanced exercise, push your hands against each other to build strength.

Land Exercise 19.
5-Count Arm Raises

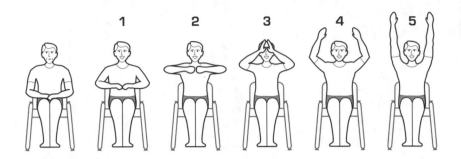

PURPOSE

This exercise improves your upper-body balance and increases ROM in your shoulders and arms.

STARTING POSITION

Sit erect with your hands in your lap.

ACTION

1. Raise both arms just below chest level with your elbows out to the sides and your hands lightly touching together.

2. With arms in same position, raise them just above shoulder level.

3. Raise your arms just above your head with your fingertips touching together.

4. Raise your arms slightly above your head with your hands spread apart.

5. Raise your arms straight up over your head.

6. Reverse the movement step-by-step, returning to the starting position.

COMMENTS

Make each move distinct, and hold that position for one second. Concentrate on maintaining balance. Use your back and abdominal muscles to prevent yourself from swaying.

Land Exercise 20.
Arm Extensions

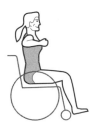 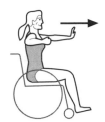 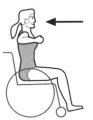 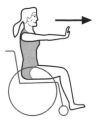

PURPOSE

This exercise improves upper-body balance; stretches the shoulder and arm muscles; and increases strength and ROM in the arms, wrists, and hands.

STARTING POSITION

Sit erect with your arms held up at shoulder level, with your elbows bent outward and your hands closed in front of your chest.

ACTION

1. Open your right hand, and slowly push your arm straight out, fully extending it. Hold this position for two to three seconds.

2. Return your hand slowly back to your chest, and close it.

3. Repeat action with your left arm.

COMMENTS

As you extend your arm, keep your hand pointing upward (as if pushing against a wall). In the beginning, you may have difficulty maintaining balance. If so, only partially extend your arm. Locate a spot in front of you in the distance. Concentrate on that spot to help maintain your balance.

Land Exercise 21.
Stomach Roll

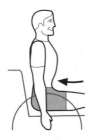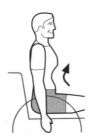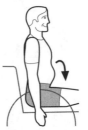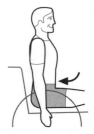

PURPOSE

This exercise stimulates and tones the abdominal muscles. It also helps peristalsis.

STARTING POSITION

Sit erect.

ACTION

Roll the abdominal muscles in a continuous wavelike motion:

1. Suck your stomach in by contracting your abdominal muscles. Pull in the lower portion of your stomach first, and then pull in the top portion.

2. Push out at the top of the stomach, and then push out toward the bottom.

3. Perform about two or three repetitions, then reverse the direction of the wave.

COMMENTS

This exercise is similar to a belly dancer's stomach roll. It will improve the function of your gastrointestinal system. Perform this exercise several times each day. At first, you may not have any control of your abdominal muscles. Keep attempting this exercise. Eventually it will produce results.

Land Exercise 22.
Tight Butt

PURPOSE

This exercise builds up the group of muscles at the base of the spine by strengthening the muscles of the buttocks (the glutei).

STARTING POSITION

Sit erect.

ACTION

1. Tighten the buttocks by contracting the gluteal muscles.

2. Hold the muscles tight for five to eight seconds.

3. Relax the muscles.

COMMENTS

The gluteus maximus (the largest gluteal muscle) is one of the largest muscles in the human body. Perform sets of repetitions of this exercise several times a day, speeding up or slowing down the exercise by changing the length of time you hold the contraction. Initially, you may not feel any results. Try to wake up the nerves and muscles. This is an isometric exercise, which builds strength by contracting muscles. As you gain control, hold the contraction for ten to fifteen seconds.

Land Exercise 23.
Hip Moves

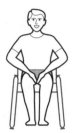 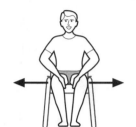 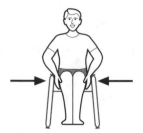

PURPOSE

This exercise stretches the lateral leg muscles (the hip abductors and hip adductors), and stimulates the nerves and muscles in the upper legs.

STARTING POSITION

Sit erect with your hands between your knees.

ACTION

1. Spread your knees apart with your hands, visualizing that the action is being done by the legs and using as much of the leg muscles as are usable.

2. Put your hands on the outside of your knees and push your legs together so the knees touch.

MINDSET

Visualize your legs moving without the help of your hands. Strain to move the legs, stimulating the nerves and muscles to wake up.

COMMENTS

You may also try placing your hands on your thighs and pushing your legs together and pulling them apart.

Land Exercise 24.
Reach Downs

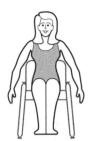 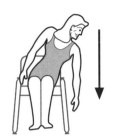 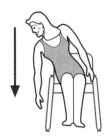

PURPOSE

This exercise improves upper-body balance and stretches and strengthens the shoulder, back, and side muscles.

STARTING POSITION

Sit erect with your arms down at your sides.

ACTION

1. Lean to the left and extend your left arm straight down. Point your head down, looking at your left hand. At the same time, raise your right shoulder up high. Let your right arm hang loose.

2. Return to the starting position.

3. Repeat this action in the opposite direction.

COMMENTS

If you have limited upper-body strength, lean over only a short distance. Use the momentum of dropping your shoulder to help you sit up. Proceed slowly, stretching out the muscles. As strength and balance improve, lean over farther.

Land Exercise 25.
Lower-Arm Raises

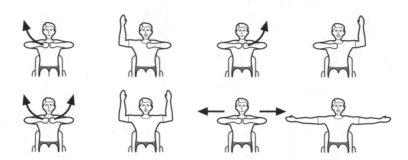

PURPOSE

This exercise strengthens the arm muscles; improves upper-body balance and coordination; and increases ROM in the shoulders, elbows, wrists, and hands.

STARTING POSITION

Sit erect with your arms held up at shoulder level, elbows bent outward, and hands closed in front of your chest.

ACTION

1. Raise your right forearm, keeping your elbow in place at shoulder level. Open your hand.
2. Return to starting position.
3. Raise your left forearm, keeping your elbow in place at shoulder level. Open your hand.
4. Return to the starting position.
5. Raise both forearms, keeping your elbows in place at shoulder level. Open your hands.
6. Return to starting position.
7. Extend both arms straight out to the sides at shoulder level. Open your hands.
8. Return to the starting position.

COMMENTS

Maintain body awareness while doing this exercise. Pay attention to coordination. Be sure to fully extend your arms, wrists, and fingers.

Land Exercise 26.
Diagonal Arm Circles

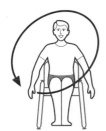 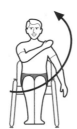 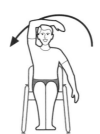 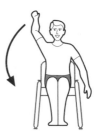

PURPOSE

This exercise improves upper-body balance and increases ROM in your shoulders.

STARTING POSITION

Sit erect with your arms down at your sides.

ACTION

Swing your right arm in a large diagonal circle:

1. Raise your right arm diagonally across your body in front of you.

2. Sweep your arm around in a large circle, raising it straight up, extending it out to the right, and returning your arm to the position in step 1.

3. Perform several repetitions, then switch sides, swinging the left arm.

COMMENTS

Concentrate on balance. Sit erect as your arm moves. At first you may need to move very slowly to prevent yourself from wobbling.

VARIATION

Perform the same exercise, circling your arms in reverse.

Land Exercise 27.
Arm Cranks

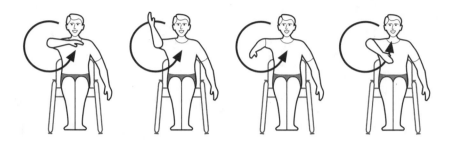

PURPOSE

This exercise improves body balance and increases ROM in the arms.

STARTING POSITION

Sit erect with your left arm down at your side and your right arm raised to shoulder level with your elbow bent outward and your forearm across your chest.

ACTION

1. Rotate your lower arm around in circles, pivoting at the elbow and keeping your upper arm out straight.
2. Perform several circular motions, then switch sides, and circle with the left arm.

COMMENTS

You may have difficulty maintaining balance at first. Begin by holding onto the wheel of your wheelchair for support with the unoccupied hand. As your balance improves, let your other arm hang down at your side.

Land Exercise 28.
Arm Circles in Front

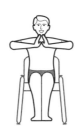 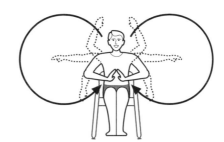

PURPOSE

This exercise improves upper-body balance and increases ROM in the neck, shoulders, and arms.

STARTING POSITION

Sit erect with your arms up at chest level, palms together in front, and your fingers pointing upward.

ACTION

Swing your arms in large circles in opposite directions.

1. Bring your hands up to about eye level, then raise your arms up over your head and then straight out to the sides.

2. As you lower your arms, point your hands down.

3. As you bring your arms back to the center, bend your elbows, and bring your hands back together.

4. Make several circles, then reverse directions—Place backs of hands together in front, with your fingers pointing down; then move your hands down, and circle out to the sides.

COMMENTS

Remove the wheelchair armrests to achieve the maximum ROM in the arms. As your hands go up, tilt your head back. As your hands go down, tilt your head down.

Land Exercise 29.
Arm Flutters

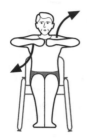 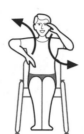 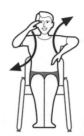

PURPOSE

This exercise improves upper-body balance and strengthens the shoulders, lower back, and abdominal muscles.

STARTING POSITION

Sit erect with your arms held up at shoulder level with your elbows bent outward and your hands closed in front of your chest.

ACTION

1. Pivoting at the elbows, rotate your arms about 45 degrees up and down. Tilt one arm up as the other arm tilts down.

2. Continue fluttering your arms and slowly extend them out straight in front of you as you move them. Open your hands.

3. Continue fluttering your arms, and slowly return to the starting position.

COMMENTS

Initially, you may not have enough upper-body strength to maintain balance. If so, keep your arms in close to your chest. As your strength improves, extend your arms out farther.

Land Exercise 30.
Twists

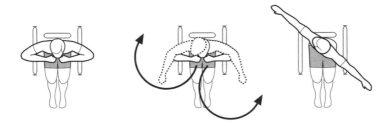

PURPOSE

This exercise improves upper-body balance. It also increases ROM in the neck, back, and arms and stretches the shoulder and lateral muscles.

STARTING POSITION

Sit erect with your arms held up at shoulder level with your elbows bent out to the side and your hands closed in front of your chest.

ACTION

1. Extend your arms straight out to the sides, open your hands, and twist your body to the left while turning your head to the left. Hold this position for three to five seconds.

2. Return to the starting position.

3. Repeat this action, turning and twisting to the right.

COMMENTS

Maintain body awareness while doing this exercise. Coordinate your arm movements. Pay attention to deep breathing. Keep your elbows at shoulder level, while lifting your diaphragm. At first, do this exercise slowly. As your balance improves, do different sets of repetitions at different speeds.

Land Exercise 31.
Push and Pull

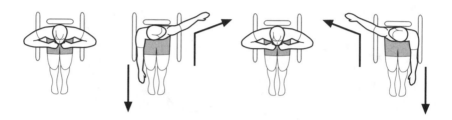

PURPOSE

This exercise improves upper-body balance and increases ROM in the shoulder and arm muscles.

STARTING POSITION

Sit erect with your arms held up at shoulder level with your elbows bent out to the sides and your hands closed in front of your chest.

ACTION

1. Slowly extend your right arm straight out in front of you with your hand open and flexed, as if pushing against a wall. At the same time, turn your head to the left, pull back with your left arm and extend it out behind you.

2. Slowly return to the starting position.

3. Repeat this exercise using opposite hands.

COMMENTS

As you reach one arm behind you, twist your body. Perform this exercise slowly. Concentrate on balance.

Land Exercise 32.
Cross-Country Skiing

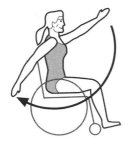 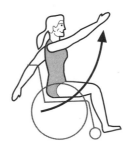

PURPOSE

This exercise improves upper-body balance, coordination, and cardio-vascular conditioning and stretches your shoulder and arm muscles.

STARTING POSITION

Sit erect with your left arm extended straight out in front of you, just above your head. Extend your right arm behind you, pointing down just a bit with both hands clenched in fists. Pretend you are gripping a ski pole in each hand.

ACTION

1. Keeping your arms straight, swoop your left arm down and behind you, while swinging your right arm up high in front.

2. Alternate, pushing your right arm down and back and your left arm forward and up.

COMMENTS

Keep your eyes on an object or an imaginary point straight ahead to maintain your balance. In the beginning, do the motions slowly and limit the distance you swing your arms. As you become more advanced, swing your arms fully to get a vigorous workout.

Land Exercise 33.
Lean Forward

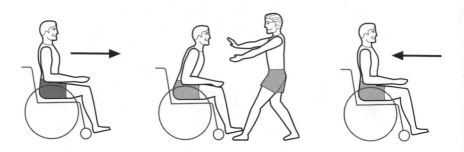

PURPOSE

This exercise improves balance and strengthens your lower-back and abdominal muscles.

STARTING POSITION

Sit erect with your arms resting on your legs. Have an assistant stand in front of you.

ACTION

1. With your chin up, slowly lean as far forward as you can without falling. Do not use your arms for support.
2. Return to the upright position.

MINDSET

Recall which muscles you used to lean forward and back. Strain to make the movements, and visualize that you are doing the exercises with full ROM, even though your movements may be slight.

COMMENTS

Initially, your assistant should place his or her hands on your shoulders as you lean forward to prevent you from falling. As you practice, judge how far you can lean on your own. As your strength improves, have the assistant stand farther away.

Land Exercise 34.
Downhill Skiing

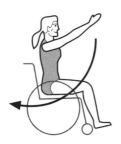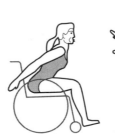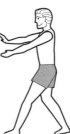

PURPOSE

This exercise improves your upper-body balance, coordination, and endurance; stretches your shoulder and arm muscles; and builds up strength in your back muscles.

STARTING POSITION

Sit erect with your arms stretched out in front of you and your hands clenched in fists.

ACTION

1. Swing both arms down and behind you, and lean forward. Keep your chin up, looking straight ahead.
2. Return to the starting position using your back muscles.

COMMENTS

In the beginning, have an assistant stand in front of you to support your body if you fall forward. Do this exercise slowly, and limit the distance you lean forward and swing your arms. As you become more advanced, lean forward farther and fully extend your arms.

VARIATION

Pretend you are chopping wood. Do this exercise with your hands together, and bring your arms down between your knees.

Land Exercise 35.
Clap Behind

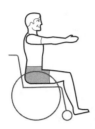 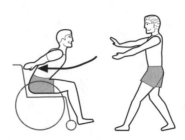 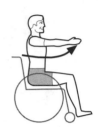

PURPOSE

This exercise improves upper-body balance and stretches your back, shoulder, and arm muscles.

STARTING POSITION

Sit erect with your arms held straight out in front of you.

ACTION

1. Lean forward and clap your hands together behind your back. Keep your chin up, looking straight ahead.

2. Return to the starting position.

COMMENTS

Depending upon the extent of your injury and your amount of muscle control, you may find it difficult to lean forward without support. Have an assistant stand in front of you to support your body if you fall forward. If your wheelchair has a large backrest, your hands may not reach together. In this case, bring your arms back as far as you can. As your muscle control improves, increase difficulty by leaning farther forward, and raising your arms up higher behind you.

Land Exercise 36.
Knee Pick-ups

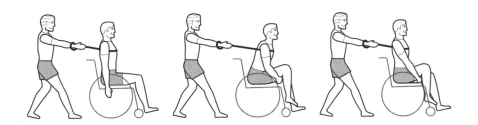

PURPOSE

This exercise wakes up the nerves in the lower legs and strengthens the arm and leg muscles.

EQUIPMENT

A strap (a belt or exercise tubing). You will need an assistant to help you with this exercise.

STARTING POSITION

Sit erect with your arms down at your sides and the strap around your chest. Have your assistant stand behind you holding the strap.

ACTION

1. Place your hands under your right leg. Lean forward and lift your knee. Your assistant will control your movements with the strap and prevent you from falling forward. Try to lift your leg with your leg muscles. Use your arms to lift only as needed.

2. Lower your leg and relax.

3. Repeat the action with your left knee.

MINDSET

Recall the muscles used to lift your knee. Stimulate those nerves! As you raise your knee, imagine that you lifted it without using your arms. In your mind, coordinate the leg movement you see with the effort it took to make it move.

COMMENTS

This is a very difficult exercise. Work on it. Be patient. It can be achieved! Initially, you will lift your leg with your arms, and the assistant will use the strap to lower and raise the trunk of your body. Program your mind to accept the motions as if you had done them without assistance. Eventually you will do it yourself.

Land Exercise 37.
Leg Kicks

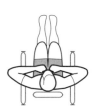 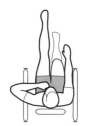 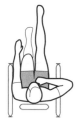

PURPOSE

This exercise stimulates the nerves, strengthens your leg muscles, and develops coordination.

STARTING POSITION

Sit erect with your hands in your lap.

ACTION

1. Attempt to kick your left leg out, and hold this position for three to five seconds. At the same time, extend your right arm in front of you.

2. Return to the starting position and relax.

3. Repeat this action with your right leg and left arm.

MINDSET

Recall the muscles used to kick out with your legs. Stimulate your nerves, and strain to make the kick. In your mind, visualize your leg out straight.

COMMENTS

Initially, you may not notice any movement, which is common. Keep trying! After a few months, have an assistant stand in front of you and watch closely for any micromovements. The weight of gravity will make movement more difficult than when performed in the water, but try, try, try!

Land Exercise 38.
Knee Lifts

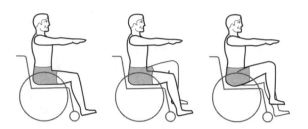

PURPOSE

This exercise stimulates the nerves and muscle function in the legs.

STARTING POSITION

Sit erect with your arms held straight out in front of you.

ACTION

1. Attempt to lift your right knee up, and hold this position for three to five seconds.

2. Bring your knee and arms back down. Relax.

3. Repeat this action with your left knee.

MINDSET

Recall the muscles used to lift your knee. Strain to lift, and visualize the knee rising up to touch your hands.

COMMENTS

Initially, you may not notice any leg movement, which is common. Continue exercising, concentrating on making it happen.

VARIATION

As you raise one knee, extend both arms out, bringing hands together above raised knee.

Land Exercise 39.
Arm Circles With Barbells

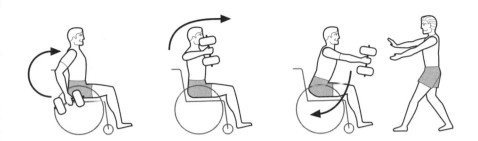

PURPOSE

This exercise improves balance, increases ROM in the arms, and strengthens the back muscles.

EQUIPMENT

Water barbells. You will need an assistant to help you with this exercise.

STARTING POSITION

Sit erect with your arms down at your sides, holding a small barbell in each hand.

ACTION

1. Circle your arms forward slowly, using a motion similar to the one used when moving the wheels on the wheelchair.

2. Perform about five to ten circular motions, then reverse direction.

COMMENTS

Your body may lean forward, throwing you off balance. In the beginning, have an assistant stand in front of you to support you. You may need to limit your arm movements to maintain balance. As your strength improves, make larger circles.

VARIATION

Use a large barbell. Perform repetitions of this exercise at different speeds.

Land Exercise 40.
Barbell Grab

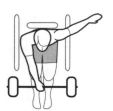 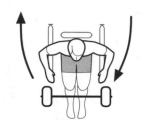 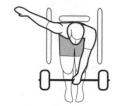

PURPOSE

This exercise improves upper-body balance, increases ROM in the arms and shoulders, and improves quickness and concentration.

EQUIPMENT

A large water barbell.

STARTING POSITION

Sit erect with your right arm stretched out behind you and your left arm held straight out in front of you with a barbell in your left hand.

ACTION

1. Quickly let go of the barbell and switch arm positions. Snatch the barbell with the right hand before it falls.

2. Repeat the exercise switching arms.

COMMENTS

Maintain body awareness while doing this exercise. Initially, you may need to limit your arm movements to maintain balance. As balance improves, perform this exercise at different speeds.

Land Exercise 41.
Barbell Twists

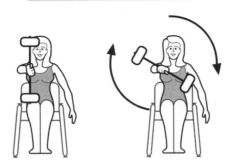

PURPOSE

This exercise improves balance, increases ROM in the arms and wrists, and strengthens the arm muscles.

EQUIPMENT

Large water barbell.

STARTING POSITION

Sit erect with your right arm extended in front of you, holding a barbell vertically in your right hand.

ACTION

1. Twist your right wrist and arm to the left as far as they will go.

2. Twist back to the right as far as your arm will go.

3. Perform about five to ten repetitions, then change hands and exercise the left arm.

COMMENTS

Maintain body awareness while doing this exercise. Pay attention to your deep breathing. Try to keep the arm at the same height as you twist. Perform sets of repetitions of this exercise at different speeds.

VARIATION

Twist the barbell using both arms. Place your hands close together in the center of bar.

Land Exercise 42.
Barbell Lift

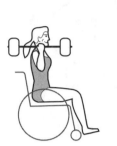 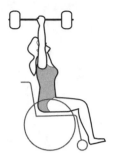

PURPOSE

This exercise improves upper-body balance and strength and increases ROM in the neck and shoulders.

EQUIPMENT

Large water barbells.

STARTING POSITION

Sit erect with barbells held horizontally in each hand at shoulder height.

ACTION

1. Push barbells straight up, fully extending the arms. Tilt your head back and look up. Inhale.

2. Lower your arms and head to starting position. Exhale.

COMMENTS

Maintain body awareness and pelvis stability throughout exercise. Concentrate on deep breathing.

Land Exercise 43.
Curls

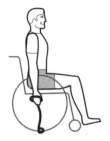 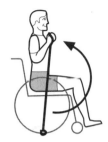

PURPOSE

This exercise strengthens the bicep muscles in the arms and the wrist muscles.

EQUIPMENT

Two-foot-long exercise tubing.

STARTING POSITION

Secure tubing to the base or wheel of your wheelchair. Sit erect with your arms down at your sides. Hold the tubing in your right hand.

ACTION

1. Raise your right hand up to shoulder level, keeping your upper arm still.
2. Return to starting position.
3. Repeat action with your left arm.

COMMENTS

Keep your upper arm stationary, moving only the lower part of your arm. If you have difficulty maintaining your balance, hold onto the wheel of your chair with your left hand. As you progress, curl both arms at the same time.

Land Exercise 44.
Triceps Extension

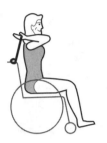 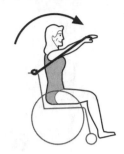

PURPOSE

This exercise strengthens the lower back, arms (triceps), and wrist muscles.

EQUIPMENT

Two-foot-long exercise tubing.

STARTING POSITION

Secure tubing to the back of your wheelchair. Sit erect. Hold the tubing in your right hand. Reach your right arm up and back over its shoulder. Hold the armrest of the wheelchair with your left hand.

ACTION

1. Keeping your upper arm still, raise your right hand up straight and bring it forward.

2. Return to the starting position.

3. Repeat this action with your left arm.

COMMENTS

Keep your upper arm stationary, moving only the lower portion of your arm.

Land Exercise 45.
Arm Raise

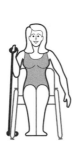 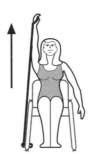

PURPOSE

This exercise strengthens the arm and shoulder muscles and increases ROM in neck.

EQUIPMENT

Two-foot-long exercise tubing.

STARTING POSITION

Secure the tubing to the side or the wheel of your wheelchair. Sit erect. With your right arm at your side bent upward at the elbow, hold the tubing in your right hand. Let your left arm hang down at your side.

ACTION

1. Raise your right arm straight up. Hold for two to three seconds. Turn your head up, following the motion of your hand, and inhale.

2. Return to the starting position and exhale while lowering your arm.

3. Repeat this action with your left arm.

COMMENTS

Keep your arms and shoulders close to the side of your head while extending your arm.

VARIATIONS

Raise both arms at same time. Turn your head alternately up, down, left, right, and straight while raising your arms.

Land Exercise 46.
Arm Circles to the Sides

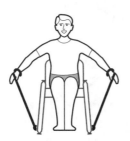 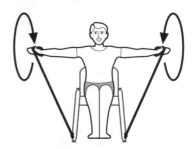

PURPOSE

This exercise strengthens the shoulder (deltoid), chest, and rib-cage muscles.

EQUIPMENT

Two-foot-long exercise tubing.

STARTING POSITION

Secure tubing at the base of your wheelchair. Sit erect with your arms fully extended at 45-degree angles from the floor, holding tubing in each hand.

ACTION

1. Rotate your arms in a forward circular motion.

2. Rotate your arms in the opposite direction.

COMMENTS

Maintain body awareness while doing this exercise. Inhale as your shoulders go up, exhale as they go down. Modify the exercise with small and large circles, performing sets of repetitions at different speeds.

Land Exercise 47.
Flying

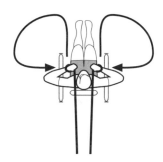

PURPOSE

This exercise strengthens the upper-back, arm, and chest muscles and improves posture.

EQUIPMENT

Twelve-foot-long exercise tubing.

STARTING POSITION

Secure tubing just above shoulder level to a post behind your wheel-chair. Sit erect with your arms up at shoulder level and your elbows bent out to the sides. With your hands centered at the top of your chest, hold the tubing in each hand. The tubing should lie on the top of your shoulders.

ACTION

1. Reach your arms straight out in front and then out to the sides.

2. Return to the starting position.

COMMENTS

Maintain body awareness while doing this exercise. Keep your elbows at shoulder level. Perform this exercise in both directions.

Land Exercise 48.
Arm Circles With Tubing

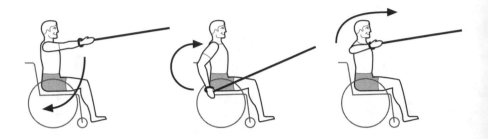

PURPOSE

This exercise strengthens your shoulder, back, abdominal, and arm muscles and improves balance and ROM in the upper body.

EQUIPMENT

Long exercise tubing.

STARTING POSITION

Secure tubing to a post three to four feet above shoulder level in front of you. Sit erect. Put your hands through loops at the ends of the tubing and extend your arms out in front of you.

ACTION

1. Make circles with your arms, pulling down and back on the tubing and then moving your arms up and around to the front in large circular motions.

2. Reverse the direction of your arm movement, circling in reverse.

VARIATIONS

Perform this exercise with your wheelchair facing the opposite direction with the tubing anchored from behind. Secure the tubing at different heights.

Land Exercise 49.
Skiing

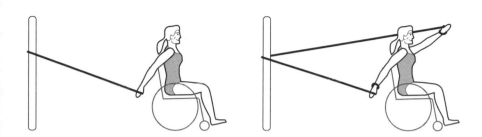

PURPOSE

This exercise develops coordination, strengthens the arm muscles, improves cardiovascular endurance, and improves deep breathing.

EQUIPMENT

Long exercise tubing.

STARTING POSITION

Secure the tubing to a post behind your wheelchair just above shoulder level. Sit erect with your arms extended behind you. Hold the tubing in both hands.

ACTION

1. Swing your left arm forward and your right arm back as if cross-country skiing.

2. Reverse arm positions.

COMMENTS

Keep your arms straight while doing this exercise.

VARIATION

Turn your chair around; so that the tubing is anchored from behind.

Land Exercise 50.
Arm Stretch With Tubing

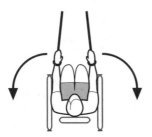 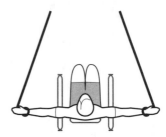

PURPOSE

This exercise strengthens the lower-back, abdominal, chest, and arm muscles; improves balance and ROM in the upper body; and improves deep breathing.

EQUIPMENT

Twelve-foot-long exercise tubing.

STARTING POSITION

Secure tubing to a post in front of you just above shoulder level. Sit erect with your arms extended in front of you holding the tubing.

ACTION

1. Spread your arms out to sides. Hold this position for three to five seconds. Inhale.

2. Return to starting position. Exhale.

COMMENTS

Work with your arms and elbows fully extended. Concentrate on deep breathing.

VARIATION

Perform the same exercise with the chair turned around so that the tubing is anchored behind you.

Land Exercise 51.
Pull Downs

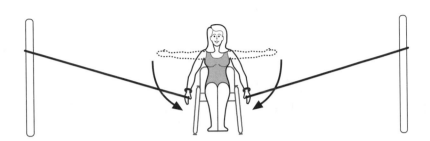

PURPOSE

This exercise strengthens the shoulder and arm muscles and improves stability and body alignment.

EQUIPMENT

Two pieces of long exercise tubing.

STARTING POSITION

Secure tubing to posts on each side of you, just above shoulder level. Sit erect holding the tubing with your arms out to the sides.

ACTION

1. Slowly pull your arms down simultaneously. Exhale.

2. Raise your arms up, elevating sideward as high as possible. Inhale.

COMMENTS

It is important to change the location of exercises: Do this exercise in the bedroom, the living room, outdoors, patio, with friends, etc. A change will keep it interesting!

Land Exercise 52.
Cross Your Chest

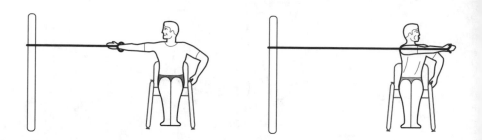

PURPOSE

This exercise strengthens the chest and arm muscles and improves stability.

EQUIPMENT

Long exercise tubing.

STARTING POSITION

Secure tubing to a post to your right, just above shoulder level. Sit erect. With your right arm extended straight out to the side, hold the tubing in that hand. Hold onto the wheel of your chair with your left hand.

ACTION

1. Pull your right arm horizontally across your chest as far as possible.

2. Return to the starting position.

COMMENTS

Pull your arm in and extend it out slowly. Keep your elbow up at shoulder level. Perform several repetitions, then turn your chair around and do the same with the left arm.

Land Exercise 53.
Hug Yourself

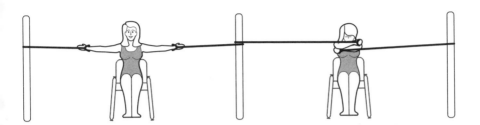

PURPOSE

This exercise strengthens the shoulder and arm muscles and improves posture, coordination, and deep breathing.

EQUIPMENT

Two pieces of long exercise tubing.

STARTING POSITION

Sit erect. Secure tubing to posts on each side of you, just above shoulder level. Extend your arms straight out to the sides while holding on to the tubing.

ACTION

1. Bring both arms in, crossing your chest (hug yourself). Tilt your head down. Exhale.

2. Return to the starting position. Inhale.

COMMENTS

With each repetition, switch the position of your top and bottom arms. Maintain body awareness. Move your arms simultaneously.

Land Exercise 54.
Breaststroke

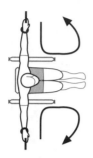 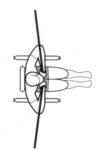 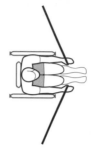 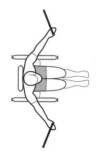

PURPOSE

This exercise strengthens the chest, shoulder, and arm muscles and improves coordination and deep breathing.

EQUIPMENT

Two pieces of long exercise tubing.

STARTING POSITION

Secure tubing at posts on each side of you, just above shoulder level. Sit erect, holding the tubing with your arms out to the sides.

ACTION

1. Draw your arms in, then push them forward, and swing them back out to the sides (a forward breaststroke).

2. Perform about one to three sets of five to ten repetitions, then reverse the action (a backward breaststroke).

COMMENTS

Pay attention to deep breathing. Inhale through your nose and blow out through pursed lips. Perform sets of repetitions at different speeds: slow, moderate pace, and fast.

PART THREE

Water
Exercises

NINE

Water Exercise Basics

Exercising in the water is the most fun and exciting part of my rehabilitation. Dr. Burdenko always uses the water with his patients to achieve results that would be much more difficult and time-consuming on the land. If you have skipped ahead and did not read Chapter 3, I recommend you take a few minutes to look it over now. Then, before you "jump" into the water, take time to review the guidelines and equipment information that follows in this part.

SAFETY ISSUES

As I have mentioned before, you do not need to know how to swim to exercise in the water. In fact, you should always wear a flotation belt or vest or other flotation device. A flotation vest will wrap around your body, providing back support, and help keep you warmer. This will help you maintain a vertical position and keep your head above water. This will also allow you to relax without needing to contract your muscles to support your body while floating.

Check with your doctor, physical therapist, or health-care practitioner before starting a water-therapy program. Make sure that you have no health problems that may prevent you from going into the water. For your own safety, as well as the safety of others, you should not enter the water if you have any of the following conditions:

- Fever or a cold.

- Open sores, wounds, or stitches.

- Urinary tract infection.

- Skin rash or a contagious condition.

- Lack of bowel or bladder control.

- Allergies or reactions to pool chemicals.

You should never be in the water alone. Always have an assistant with you—especially in the beginning. The assistant should enter the water before you, and leave after you get out. In this way, the assistant is readily available as you get accustomed to the water while you practice your balance and stability. The assistant will help you if you become fatigued and need a hand. You may also find it useful to have your assistant stay out of the water to observe your exercises and give you feedback to help you maintain body awareness.

The temperature of the water is another factor to consider. The ideal water temperature for rehabilitation is 85° to 90°F. Warm water temperature helps relax the muscles. If you are working at a higher level of conditioning and doing some aerobic workouts, it may be better if the water is a little cooler. In any case, you do not want to get a chill from working in the water. If you start to get cold, you may need to shorten the time you spend in the water. Because I am paraplegic and therefore cannot tell when I am getting a chill until it is too late, I need to have an assistant check my skin temperature from time to time.

JACUZZI

Some pools also offer a Jacuzzi. There are pros and cons associated with the use of Jacuzzis. On the plus side, the hot bubbling water will relax the muscles and help increase circulation. This may feel good if you get a little chilled while exercising in the pool. On the minus side, the heat may make you faint, and the increased circulation may raise your blood pressure. If you are paralyzed or have loss of feelings, you may not be able to judge when you have stayed in the Jacuzzi too long. If you find a Jacuzzi to your liking, use it under the guidance of your physical therapist or health-care professional. Periodically, have your blood pressure checked before and after you use the Jacuzzi to see how your heart responds to the heat.

EQUIPMENT

Just like a surgeon needs more than one knife to operate, you will need an appropriate variety of exercise equipment to help you achieve the maximum benefit from your workouts. There are a few specific items that you will need to perform the exercises: a flotation vest or belt, water barbells, a kickboard, and exercising tubing. Additional items that can be helpful to your rehabilitation and conditioning are listed in this section as well. The main consideration in selecting equipment for water exercise is safety. You need to choose equipment that is appropriate for your present physical condition and easy for you to use. Your physical therapist or health-care professional should help you make the selection.

All equipment for the water exercises should float or be mounted securely in place. If an item sinks, you may be inclined to retrieve it, which may cause problems.

The Flotation Vest

The most important equipment you will use in the water is the flotation vest or belt. In recent years, this equipment has been designed specifically for exercising in the water. There are a variety of styles on the market offering different degrees of buoyancy. First and foremost, it must keep you afloat, making it completely safe to be in the water. Secondly, it will help support your body in the vertical position while exercising, which is an essential part of the Burdenko Method.

The flotation device should be in good condition. If you purchase a new piece of equipment, adjust the straps and fasteners so it fits snugly without being too tight. If you select used equipment, make sure that there are no cracks in the flotation material, and ensure that the straps and fasteners are not worn out. Do not use a flotation device that is too small or oversized. It should fit properly.

A vest allows the center of buoyancy to be high on the body, providing good stability, which is important for most wheelchair users. (See Figure 9.1 at right.) Additionally, a vest helps retain body warmth, which may be helpful if the water temperature is cool. The Wet Vest is the most popular flotation vest on the market. Its unique patented features provide buoyancy and support with a minimal amount of interference, allowing unrestricted movement in the water.

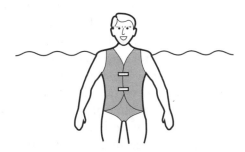

Figure 9.1. The flotation vest.

The Flotation Belt and Cuffs

In the advanced stages of your rehabilitation, you may prefer using a flotation belt. When choosing a belt, make sure that it is the type that distributes buoyancy around the whole body, allowing you to maintain the vertical position in the water. A good example is the Hydro-Fit belt and cuffs. (See

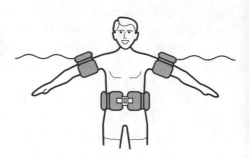

Figure 9.2. The flotation belt and cuffs.

Figure 9.2, right.) It has a modular design, consisting of a series of flotation pockets fastened together. Flotation material can be added or removed from each pocket to adjust the buoyancy. It can be worn as a belt, or as smaller cuffs on the arms or ankles.

Water Barbells

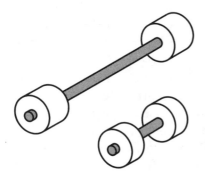

Figure 9.3. Water barbells.

Water barbells are made from a plastic tube with floats at each end. (See Figure 9.3, left.) The barbells are used to provide resistance when held underwater and support when they are placed under your body. You will need two large barbells and two small barbells. The large barbell is 30 inches long and is ideal for sitting upon, for holding with one arm or both arms, and for placing under your ankles when lying on your back, to keep your legs afloat.

The small barbell is just large enough to be held in one hand. Some manufacturers make barbells with removable floats. These will let you add or decrease the buoyancy by changing the number of floats.

Floats come in two different styles—circular and triangular. The circular floats offer the same resistance when pushed or pulled and are easy to use. The triangular style lets you vary the resistance by pushing either the point or the flat side through the water. The triangular style may be harder to use if you do not have adequate hand strength. In pushing and pulling exercises, you need to rotate the barbell each time you change direction to get the same resistance. When exercising in one direction, you need to be able to hold the bar to prevent it from rotating.

The Kickboard

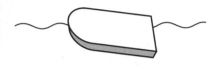

Figure 9.4. The kickboard.

A kickboard is a piece of Styrofoam or other flotation material $1\frac{1}{4}$ to 2 inches thick. (See Figure 9.4, left.) Their sizes come in 12 inches by 18 inches and 12 inches by 24 inches. As the name implies, the kickboard was originally designed to be held with both hands out in front as you practice kicking. I use the kickboard to provide resistance during my exercises, pushing it and pulling it through the water. The amount of resistance can be varied by laying it flat or turning it on its side. The kickboard can also be used to improve balance when it is held underwater with one hand, or when used for sitting and standing.

Push-Up Bars

Push-up bars are common items found in sporting-goods stores and department stores in the weightlifting section. (See Figure 9.5, right.) They were originally designed to be used while doing pushups, but they are very useful for wheelchair users in helping prepare for exercises in the water.

I use push-up bars whenever I transfer between my wheelchair and the ground. The push-up bar helps

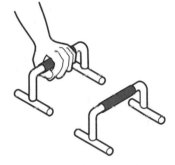

Figure 9.5. Push-up bars.

extend my arm reach, making it easier to reach the ground. When sitting on the ground, the push-up bars make it easy to lift your bottom and move. It is much easier than sliding without them.

A note of caution: Push-up bars require good strength in your wrists. When your arm is extended at an angle to the ground and you shift your weight, the push-up bar has a tendency to tip over (in the same direction you shift your weight), so your hands and wrists must be strong enough to handle the load.

Exercise Tubing

This is the same tubing that is used for land exercises. (See Figure 9.6 on page 156.) It is useful in the water in several ways. Just as with land exercises, tubing can be used to add resistance to increase the

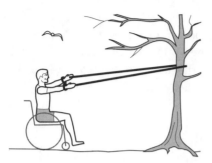

Figure 9.6. Exercise tubing.

difficulty of exercises. It is extremely useful in many exercises where the tubing is attached from the arms to the legs. Arm movements in the water will then pull the legs along. This leg movement helps to stimulate the nerves and muscle tissue.

Tubing will wear out with use. Always inspect the tubing and replace it when it has cracks or shows any sign of wear.

Adjustable Rings

I did not use adjustable rings in my program; however, Dr. Burdenko recommends them for use in the pool. Adjustable rings suspend from the ceiling. (See Figure 9.7, right.) They can be raised and lowered to different heights above and below the water. They are very useful for keeping the body extended and rigid and for developing upper-body strength. The rings can be used for pushups and pull-ups from the horizontal position and chin-ups from the vertical position.

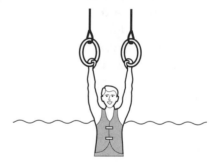

As you advance in your recovery, you can stand with your feet in the rings under the water and perform forward, backward, and sideways splits. The higher the rings are raised out of the water, the more effort it will take to perform the exercises.

Figure 9.7. Adjustable rings.

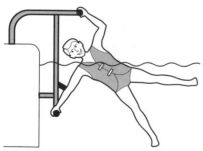

Figure 9.8. The Water Workout Station.

The Water Workout Station

A Water Workout Station can provide a gym setting in the water. Aquatrend makes a portable unit that simply hangs over the edge of a pool. It consists of a stainless-steel framework with grips for the hands and feet. (See Figure 9.8, left.) It also has a platform that swings down below the surface for sitting and performing exercises. It can be used for a variety of activities, including pull-ups, lateral raises, abdominal crunches, leg curls, and many more.

The Pool Lift

I transfer into and out of the pool without the use of a lift; however, a pool lift may be a necessity for some wheelchair users. There are electric, hand-operated, and water-powered models. The lift may allow the user to be raised and lowered while seated or lying down, depending upon his or her physical condition. (See Figure 9.9, right.) Some units can be operated by the user, and others require an attendant. Lifts are designed for in-ground, as well as above-ground, pools.

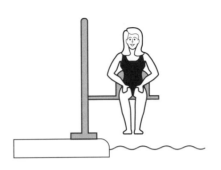

Figure 9.9. The pool lift.

GETTING IN AND OUT OF THE WATER

Remember, water exercises can be performed anywhere there is water, for example, in a lake. You can transfer out of your chair onto the sand and then down to the water. I generally transfer in stages. First, I go to a lower beach chair, and then down to the sand. I make my way along the sand using push-up bars to lift my bottom as I slide over and move along.

Most facilities designed for water therapy have a pool with a special lift for the handicapped. You transfer from the wheelchair into the seat of the lift, and your assistant will operate the controls and lower you gently into the water. You may not have access to a lift all the time. This should not restrict you from getting in and out of the pool. The technique you use will depend upon your physical capabilities. The following is the technique that Dr. Burdenko designed for me. (Note: I will describe the actions transferring to my right side. From time to time, you should alternate sides to make your transfer balanced.)

Before entering the water, put on your flotation vest or belt. Position yourself at the corner of the pool. Slide forward, letting the lower portion of your legs down into the water.

Place a pool lounge chair on the right side of the wheelchair. If you do not have a lounge chair, use a stool or low chair, where the height of the seat is about halfway between the floor and the wheel-chair seat. To the right of the lounge chair, place a seat cushion on the floor. Position the wheelchair against the lounge chair at a 45-degree angle. (See Figure 9.10, below.) This makes it easier to slide your bottom out of the wheelchair without rubbing against the wheel on the side. (My wheelchair has removable legs. Before positioning the wheelchair at an angle, I remove the right wheelchair leg. When the wheelchair leg is removed, I put my right foot on top of my left foot so it does not drag on the ground.)

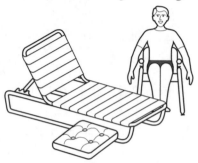

Figure 9.10. Transferring from the wheelchair to the floor—starting position.

Slide your buttocks over to the edge of the wheelchair seat. Remove the right armrest from your wheelchair. Swing your right leg over in front of the lounge chair. With your left hand, grip onto the wheelchair armrest for support. Lean over to the right, and put your right hand down onto the lounge chair. Then, pushing with both arms, slide sideways down into the lounge chair.

Swing your left leg over in front of the lounge chair. Then swing both legs to the right in front of the seat cushion. Scoot your bottom over to the right edge of the lounge chair. Place your left hand down onto the lounge chair next to your buttocks. Lean over and place your right hand onto the far edge of the seat cushion. (If you have difficulty reaching down to the cushion, use a push-up bar to extend your reach.) Pushing up with both arms, slide sideways down onto the seat cushion. (See Figure 9.11, right.)

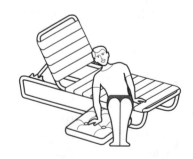

Figure 9.11. Transferring from lounge chair to floor.

Using a push-up bar in each hand to raise your bottom up off the floor, transfer over to the corner of the pool. This may take several moves. Slide your legs over with each move. (See Figure 9.12 on page 159.)

With your right hand, hold onto the right edge of the pool. With your left hand, hold onto the left edge of the pool. Lean forward, moving your hands out along the edges of the pool. Do a pushup,

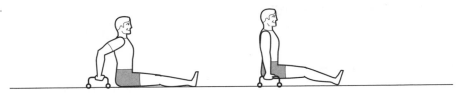

Figure 9.12. Moving along the floor using push-up bars.

raising your bottom up and out over the water. Slowly lower yourself into the pool. (See Figure 9.13, below.)

The technique for getting out of the pool is the reverse. Back up into the corner, facing into the pool. Bend your elbows up high and place your hands on either edge of the pool. Do a pushup, leaning slightly forward, and raise your bottom up out of the water and onto the edge. Then scoot back onto the seat cushion. Remove your flotation vest and dry off with a towel. You deserve a break.

If this technique does not work for you, be creative! There is always a way to get into the water.

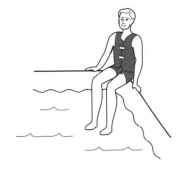

Figure 9.13. Entering the pool.

Water Exercises

LARGE BARBELL EXERCISES

1. Forward Stretch
2. Side Stretch
3. Horizontal Stretch
4. Stand up From Lying on Back
5. Angels in the Snow
6. Upright Push-Pulls
7. Prone Push-Pulls
8. Parallel Barbell Push Downs
9. Push Down With a Single Barbell
10. Jumping Jacks
11. The American Crawl
12. Walking With Barbells
13. Breaststroke on Back With Barbell
14. Back Sway With Barbells 1
15. Back Sway With Barbells 2
16. Twist With Barbells
17. Jump and Walk With Barbells
18. Sit-ups With Barbell Under the Knees
19. Barbell Sitting While Holding the Wall

LARGE BARBELL EXERCISES (continued)

20. Barbell Sitting
21. Sit and Swim
22. Upright Barbell Balancing
23. Sit up and Over
24. Knee Raises With Barbells at the Sides
25. Roll-Overs
26. Straddling the Barbell
27. Swim and Step

SMALL BARBELL EXERCISES

28. Jog in Place With Small Barbells
29. Side Swings With Small Barbells
30. Stretch-Outs With Small Barbells
31. Arm Swings With Small Barbells
32. Leg Kicks With Small Barbells
33. Small Barbell Pass
34. Barbell Boxing

EXERCISES WITH NO EQUIPMENT

35. Walking
36. Upright Breaststroke
37. Side Stroke
38. Balancing on Your Side
39. Pushups in the Corner
40. Leg Lifts From the Corner
41. Backward Leg Lifts in the Corner
42. Knee Raises at the Wall
43. Knee Raises in the Corner
44. Crawling up in the Corner
45. Horizontal Stretch in the Corner
46. Upright Twist and Turn
47. Stand up at the Wall
48. Circle Kick
49. Side Step
50. Horizontal Stretching at the Ladder
51. Turning Along the Wall
52. Catch Your Knee

KICKBOARD EXERCISES

53. Balance With the Kickboard
54. Vertical Kickboard Strokes
55. Kickboard Twist
56. Push to the Rear
57. Prone Pushups

TUBING EXERCISES

58. Backward Breaststroke
59. Swim With Short Tubing
60. Swim With Attached Tubing

Water Exercise 1.
Forward Stretch

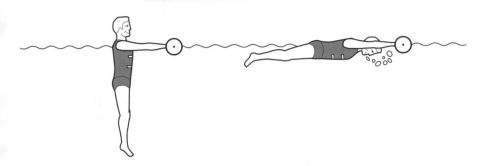

PURPOSE

This exercise stretches the neck and shoulders, works on deep breathing, and strengthens the back and abdominal muscles.

EQUIPMENT

Large barbell, flotation vest.

STARTING POSITION

Float vertically. Hold a large barbell with your arms extended out in front.

ACTION

1. Lean forward with arms stretched out in front of you and lie face down in the water. Exhale into the water.

2. Hold this position for 2 to 3 seconds. Raise your head out of the water and inhale deeply. Exhale with your face down in the water.

3. Return to the starting position.

MINDSET

Picture your body and legs in one straight line. Stretch your legs and flex your feet. Tighten the muscles in your buttocks. Visualize holding your legs together or separating them.

COMMENTS

It is important to exhale face down in the water. This will increase
your lung strength and capacity. Practice taking several deep breaths.

When lying face down in the water with your arms stretched out
in front of you, it may be difficult to lift your torso out of the water to
return to the vertical position. At first, it may be easier to roll over on
your back and then lean forward to sit up and return to the vertical
position; however, keep trying to lift yourself up from the face-down
position. This requires strength in your abdomen and lower back.
Use your head and upper-body muscles to lift. Help with your arms
by pushing down on the barbell. Once you have mastered this, concentrate on swinging your legs down as you lean back.

Water Exercise 2.
Side Stretch

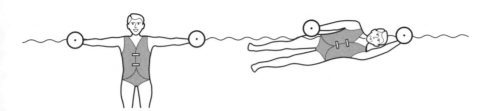

PURPOSE

This exercise stretches the shoulder and back muscles and improves balance and trunk control.

EQUIPMENT

Large barbells, flotation vest.

STARTING POSITION

Float vertically in the water, with arms out straight to sides holding barbells in each hand.

ACTION

1. Lie on your left side with your arms extended. Balance on your side for 5 to 10 seconds.

2. Return to the upright position.

3. Do the same on your right side.

MINDSET

When lying on your side, visualize your legs out straight and raised to the surface.

COMMENTS

A firm grip on the barbells will help you maintain your balance on your side. As you progress, use your body to maintain your balance and release your grip, letting your hands rest on the barbells. Breathe deeply.

Water Exercise 3.
Horizontal Stretch

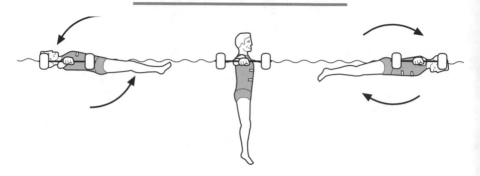

PURPOSE

This exercise teaches you how to go from one position to another.

EQUIPMENT

Large barbells, flotation vest.

STARTING POSITION

Float vertically in the water with your arms out to the sides holding a barbell in each hand.

ACTION

1. Lean forward and lie face down in the water. Exhale into the water.

2. Sit up and return to the upright vertical position.

3. Lean back and lie flat on your back.

4. Return to the starting position.

MINDSET

When lying flat, visualize your legs out straight, raised to the surface.

COMMENTS

Initially, movement will come from your arms and shoulders. As you progress, use your abdominal, neck, and trunk muscles.

Water Exercise 4.
Stand up From Lying on Back

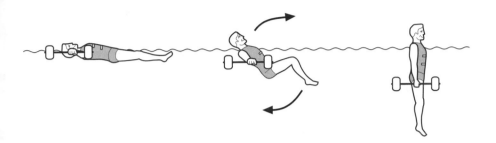

PURPOSE

This exercise strengthens the abdominal and back muscles and improves balance.

EQUIPMENT

Large barbells, flotation vest.

STARTING POSITION

Lie on your back in the water with your arms extended out to the sides with large barbells in each hand.

ACTION

1. Lunge forward, coming to the vertical position. With your arms fully extended, maintain vertical balance.
2. Return to the starting position.

MINDSET

Imagine that you can lean forward and stand up straight. Picture stretching your legs and flexing your feet, and feel the hamstrings tighten.

COMMENTS

This exercise is intended to strengthen the chest, back, and abdomen. Most people in wheelchairs have weak abdominal and gluteal muscles. At first, you will need to use your arms to help push yourself forward. As your strength improves, rely less on your arms and more on your abdominal muscles.

Water Exercise 5.
Angels in the Snow

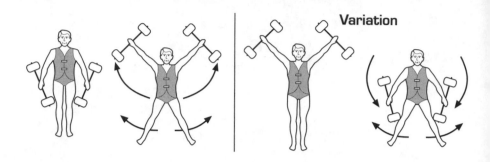

Variation

PURPOSE

This exercise stretches the shoulder and back muscles and stimulates the leg muscles and breathing.

EQUIPMENT

Large barbells, flotation vest.

STARTING POSITION

Lie on your back. With your arms at your sides, hold a barbell in each hand.

ACTION

1. Spread your legs apart. Swing your arms out to the sides and up above your head. Inhale. Hold for 5 seconds.

2. Return to the starting position. Exhale.

MINDSET

Remember how it used to feel to move the legs. Imagine your legs moving.

COMMENTS

Concentrate on extending your legs out straight and spreading them to the side. Don't hold your breath.

VARIATION 1

As your arms go up, bring your legs together. As you bring your arms down, spread your legs apart.

VARIATION 2

Perform this exercise lying face down in the water.

Water Exercise 6.
Upright Push-Pulls

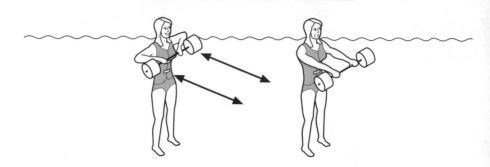

PURPOSE

This exercise stretches the shoulder and back muscles and strengthens the arm muscles.

EQUIPMENT

Large barbell, flotation vest.

STARTING POSITION

Remain vertical. Hold the barbell with both hands at shoulder width in front of your chest.

ACTION

1. Push the barbell out straight. Maintain your balance, holding your body upright.
2. Return to the starting position.

COMMENTS

Push and pull the barbell on the surface, using the water to create a gentle resistance. Begin slowly at first. As you become accustomed to this exercise, push and pull vigorously. Splash the water and have fun! Remember to breathe deeply.

Water Exercise 7.
Prone Push-Pulls

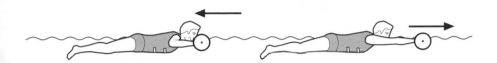

PURPOSE

This exercise stretches the shoulder and arm muscles and works on breathing and balance.

EQUIPMENT

Large barbell, flotation vest.

STARTING POSITION

Lie face down (prone) with your arms extended in front of you. Hold the barbell with both hands at shoulder width.

ACTION

1. Pull the barbell into your chest. Inhale.

2. Push the barbell out straight in front of you. Exhale.

COMMENTS

Push and pull the barbell through the water fully extending your arms, keeping your elbows straight. Begin slowly at first. As you become accustomed to this exercise, push and pull, vigorously splashing the water.

Water Exercise 8.
Parallel Barbell Push Downs

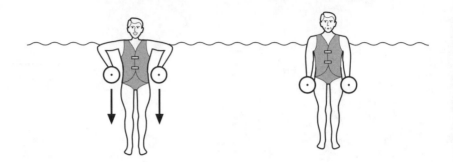

PURPOSE

This exercise stretches the shoulder and back muscles, strengthens the arms, improves balance, and helps you maintain proper body alignment.

EQUIPMENT

Large barbells, flotation vest.

STARTING POSITION

Float vertically in the water. Hold a barbell in each hand. Bend your elbows and bring the barbells in close to your sides.

ACTION

1. Push the barbells straight down. Maintain body balance.

2. Return to the starting position.

COMMENTS

This exercise can be performed slowly, concentrating on balance. It can also be performed pumping up and down vigorously to strengthen the muscles in the upper arms.

Water Exercise 9.
Push Down With a Single Barbell

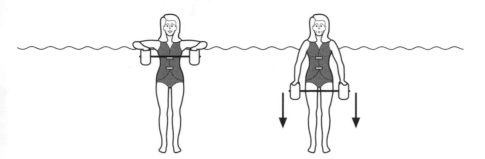

PURPOSE

This exercise improves upper-body balance, strengthens the arm and shoulder muscles, and improves ROM.

EQUIPMENT

Large barbell, flotation vest.

STARTING POSITION

Float vertically in the water. Hold the large barbell at chest level, with your hands on top of the floats.

ACTION

1. Push the barbell straight down. Maintain body balance. Hold this position for 5 seconds.

2. Return to the starting position slowly, raising the arms while maintaining balance.

COMMENTS

As you exercise and build up strength, make it more difficult by changing the starting position—move the barbell out in front of your body, a little at a time.

Water Exercise 10.
Jumping Jacks

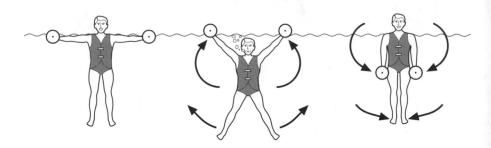

PURPOSE

This exercise improves balance, coordination, strength, and flexibility; strengthens the arm muscles; and stimulates the legs.

EQUIPMENT

Large barbells, flotation vest.

STARTING POSITION

Float vertically with your arms straight out to the sides with a barbell in each hand.

ACTION

1. Swing your arms out and up. Inhale deeply. Your body will temporarily dip farther into the water. As it does, spread your legs apart.

2. Swing your arms back down. Exhale as you come up. Bring your legs together.

MINDSET

Visualize your arms and legs moving in and out in coordination. Concentrate on sending the signal from your brain, and picture it traveling down through the nerves, stimulating the muscles in your legs.

COMMENTS

Pay special attention to breathing, coordination, and remaining vertical.

Water Exercise 11.
The American Crawl

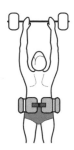 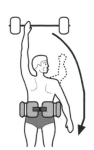 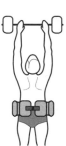 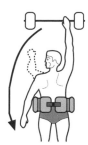

PURPOSE

This exercise stretches and strengthens the upper body.

EQUIPMENT

Large barbell, flotation belt or flotation vest.

STARTING POSITION

Lie on your stomach. Grasp a large barbell with your arms out straight in front of you.

ACTION

1. Stroke through the water with your right arm, bringing it down and back to side. Turn your head to the right and inhale.

2. Bring your right arm forward on top of the water, and grasp the barbell. Put your face down into the water and exhale.

3. Repeat steps 1 and 2 using your left arm. Turn your head left to inhale.

MINDSET

Imagine your legs kicking as your arms stroke.

COMMENTS

Concentrate on breathing and kicking your legs up and down.

Water Exercise 12.
Walking With Barbells

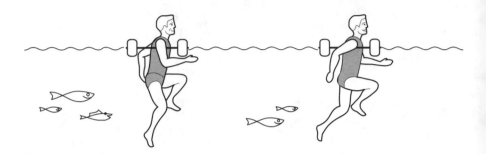

PURPOSE

This exercise strengthens the arms, stimulates the legs, and improves arm and leg coordination.

EQUIPMENT

Large barbells, flotation vest.

STARTING POSITION

Float vertically with a barbell under each armpit.

ACTION

1. In very distinct movements, take steps as if walking, swinging your arms down along your sides.

2. Coordinate your arm and leg movements. As you bring your left arm forward, step out with your right foot. As you bring your right arm forward, step out with left foot .

3. Practice the same exercise in reverse. Walk backwards.

MINDSET

If you never ask your body to walk, it won't happen. Think about how it feels to walk. Imagine that your legs work. Imagine your legs moving.

COMMENTS

Concentrate on stepping forward with one leg and pulling back on the other leg. Do not cup your hands or use them as paddles. Let your arms and legs do the work.

Water Exercise 13.
Breaststroke on Back With Barbell

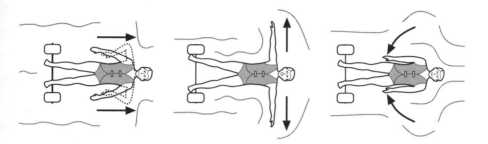

PURPOSE

This exercise strengthens the upper body, improves pelvic stability, and stimulates function in the joints of the legs and feet.

EQUIPMENT

Large barbell, flotation vest.

STARTING POSITION

Lie on your back with your legs spread apart and the barbell under the heels of your feet. Keep your feet close to the Styrofoam floats of the barbell. Let your arms hang straight down at your sides.

ACTION

1. Bring your arms up alongside your body, bending your elbows.

2. Extend your arms straight out to the sides.

3. Cup your hands and swing your arms down to sides.

4. Concentrate on holding the barbell with your heels.

MINDSET

Imagine pushing out against the Styrofoam floats with your feet.

COMMENTS

To position the barbell, start from a sitting position. Push the barbell under your legs and slide it down to your ankles. It is common for the barbell to slide off as you exercise. Even though you may not feel anything, picture your ankles working in your mind, with your heels holding the barbell in position and your feet pressed against the Styrofoam.

Water Exercise 14.
Back Sway With Barbells 1

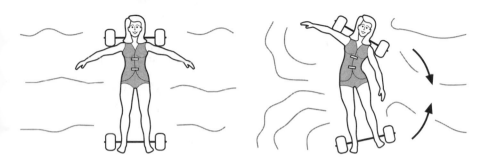

PURPOSE

This exercise stretches the upper-body and side muscles, works on pelvic stability, and stimulates the thigh muscles.

EQUIPMENT

Large barbells, flotation vest.

STARTING POSITION

Lie on your back. Position one barbell under your neck and the other under your ankles. Spread your legs apart.

ACTION

1. Bend your body to the left. Reach your left arm down to your hip and bring your right arm up. Swing your legs to the left. Feel the muscles stretch along your right side. Hold this position for 3 to 5 seconds.

2. Repeat this action on the right side.

COMMENTS

Concentrate on moving your legs and hips. It may take some practice to position the barbell under your ankles. Start from a sitting position. Push the barbell under your legs and slide it down under your ankles.

Water Exercise 15.
Back Sway With Barbells 2

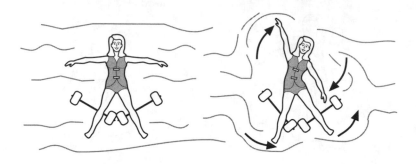

PURPOSE

This exercise improves flexibility and coordination and stretches the upper-body and side muscles.

EQUIPMENT

Large barbells, flotation vest.

STARTING POSITION

Lie on your back with your arms held out to the sides. Place a barbell under each knee.

ACTION

1. Sway to the left. Bring your left arm down to the side, and raise your right arm out and up above your shoulder. Feel the muscles stretch along your right side.

2. Now reverse the direction and sway to the right.

COMMENTS

Pay attention to your breathing and the coordination of the movement of your arms and legs.

Water Exercise 16.
Twist With Barbells

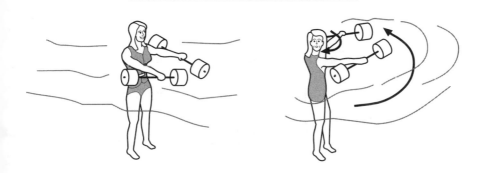

PURPOSE

This exercise increases ROM and strength in the upper body, and flexes the lateral muscles.

EQUIPMENT

Large barbells, flotation vest.

STARTING POSITION

Float vertically with your arms extended in front of you with a barbell in each hand.

ACTION

1. Rotate both arms to the left. At the same time, turn your head and your body to the right.

2. Reverse directions. Rotate both arms to the right and twist your body and head to the left.

COMMENTS

Proceed gently at first. As you gain more body control, perform this exercise vigorously. Splash and have fun! Keep your chin up, and practice deep breathing.

Water Exercise 17.
Jump and Walk With Barbells

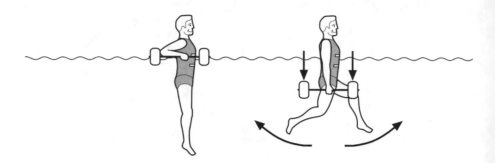

PURPOSE

This exercise stimulates leg function and improves upper-body balance, coordination, and strength.

EQUIPMENT

Large barbells, flotation vest.

STARTING POSITION

Float vertically. Hold the barbells close to your armpits.

ACTION

1. Push the barbells straight down. Move your left leg in front of you and your right leg behind you. Maintain your balance, staying upright in the water.

2. Bend your elbows, and return to the starting position.

3. Repeat this action, switching the positions of your legs.

MINDSET

Concentrate on waking up the nerves and muscles. Imagine your legs moving in the water as if you were walking.

COMMENTS

Perform this exercise at different speeds.

Water Exercise 18.
Barbell Sitting While Holding the Wall

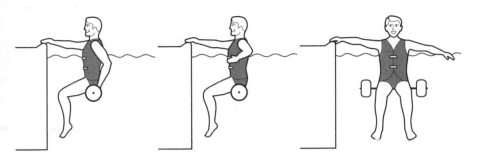

PURPOSE

This exercise improves balance and pelvic stability and strengthens the arm, wrist, back, chest, and abdominal muscles.

EQUIPMENT

Large barbell, flotation vest.

STARTING POSITION

Float vertically. Hold the wall of the pool with one hand and the large barbell in the other.

ACTION

1. Push the barbell below the surface and position it under your bottom.

2. Let go of the barbell. Sit upright and maintain your balance.

3. Hold the wall with one hand. Swing your body away from the wall. Use your free hand to help position yourself and maintain balance.

4. Return to starting position.

5. Repeat this action facing the other direction.

MINDSET

As you sit, imagine feeling the pressure of the barbell pushing up against your bottom. Picture your body being able to move slightly forward and backward and side to side to maintain your balance.

COMMENTS

This may seem like a simple exercise, but it actually requires the coordination of many muscles. In the beginning, it may be difficult to sit on the barbell. Your arms may be weak, and positioning the barbell will take some practice. The barbell may not stay in place, but stay with it, and as the weeks progress, to your surprise, the barbell will eventually stay in place.

You may need to use both hands to position the barbell. Then hold the wall for stability and practice balancing until the barbell stays in place. Balance for 10, 15, 20, and finally 30 seconds. When you have mastered this, swing out away from the wall. Maintain your balance as you move through the water. Swing back in, change hands and swing back out to the other side.

This exercise took me months to accomplish. Although I could not feel my abdominal or lower-back muscles, I somehow managed to use them to maintain my balance. This exercise really helped me believe that I was able to regain control of paralyzed muscles.

Water Exercise 19.
Barbell Sitting

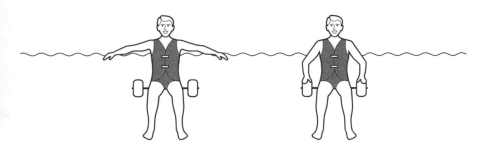

PURPOSE

This exercise improves balance and strengthens the arms, wrists, back, chest, and abdomen.

EQUIPMENT

Large barbell, flotation vest.

STARTING POSITION

Float vertically. Hold a large barbell in one hand.

ACTION

1. While sitting, push the barbell under your bottom. Use both hands to position the barbell if necessary.

2. Maintain your balance with your neck and back straight.

3. Place your hands on the Styrofoam floats of the barbell beneath the surface and maintain balance.

4. Return to starting position.

MINDSET

Imagine you are floating in a canoe, controlling your balance with your body position.

COMMENTS

This exercise is a lot of fun. It will take practice and patience. First, balance with your hands on the surface for 10, 15, 20, and finally 30 seconds. Then practice balancing with your hands on the floats. This is more difficult and will stimulate the abdominal and back muscles.

Water Exercise 20.
Sit-ups With a Barbell Under the Knees

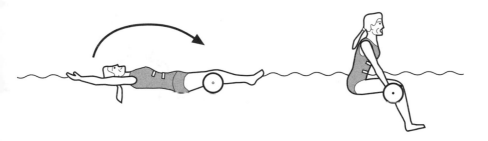

PURPOSE

This exercise strengthens the abdominal and back muscles.

EQUIPMENT

Large barbell, flotation vest.

STARTING POSITION

Lie on your back. Place the barbell under your knees. Extend your arms out over your head.

ACTION

1. Swing your arms up and stretch forward. Bend at the waist and lean forward.

2. Sit up and hold the barbell with your hands.

3. Return to the starting position.

COMMENTS

Depending upon the level of your injury, you may or may not have control of your abdominal muscles in the beginning. Use your arms for leverage, and lunge forward. As you practice this exercise, concentrate on using your abdominal muscles.

Water Exercise 21.
Sit and Swim

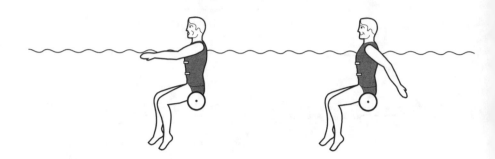

PURPOSE

This exercise improves balance and pelvic stability and strengthens the arm, back, and chest muscles.

EQUIPMENT

Large barbell, flotation vest.

STARTING POSITION

Sit on the large barbell.

ACTION

1. Use actions similar to a breaststroke from a seated position to move forward. Stretch both arms in front of you and sweep them both back behind you under the water, maintaining your balance.

2. Reverse this action to move backwards.

MINDSET

Think about your posture. Mimic your arm motions with your legs.

COMMENTS

Attempt this exercise only after you have mastered "Barbell Sitting While Holding the Wall" (see page 181). Use rhythmic strokes. Swim at different speeds.

Water Exercise 22.
Upright Barbell Balancing

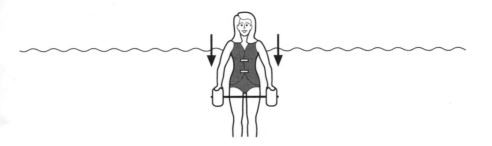

PURPOSE

This exercise improves balance and strengthens the arm, wrist, back, and abdominal muscles.

EQUIPMENT

Large barbell, flotation vest.

STARTING POSITION

Float vertically. Place your hands on top of the barbell Styrofoam floats.

ACTION

1. Slowly push the barbell down until your arms are fully extended.

2. Hold this position, and maintain your vertical balance for 3 to 4 seconds.

3. Slowly bend your elbows and return to the starting position.

COMMENTS

Maintain body awareness. Keep the barbell level. Do not let it tip to either side. Raising and lowering the barbell slowly strengthens the arms, improves coordination, and helps improve balance. Once your arms are fully extended, concentrate on maintaining your balance using your upper body. Use your torso to shift your weight instead of moving your arms. This will stimulate the abdominal and lower-back muscles.

Water Exercise 23.
Sit up and Over

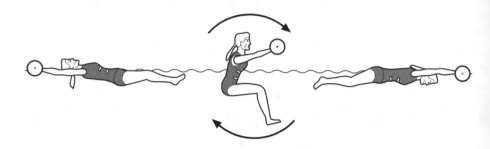

PURPOSE

This exercise improves balance and strengthens the back and abdominal muscles.

EQUIPMENT

Large barbell, flotation vest.

STARTING POSITION

Lie on your back holding the barbell with both hands, arms extended over your head.

ACTION

1. Lunge forward, sit up, and then lie on your stomach.

2. Hold this position, bringing your legs out straight for 3 to 4 seconds.

3. Roll over and resume the starting position.

MINDSET

As you use your upper body, concentrate on moving your legs to control this movement. Picture them going down through the water together. Try to awaken the muscles, and strain to make your legs move. Feel your nerves tingle.

COMMENTS

Initially, you will use your arms and the barbell's momentum to lunge forward. As you progress, concentrate on using your abdominal and back muscles. Rely less on the use of your arms.

VARIATION

Instead of rolling over to the starting position, attempt to lean back, going from lying on your stomach to lying on your back without using your arm muscles. I found this very difficult. It requires a fair amount of strength in the abdominal and back muscles.

Water Exercise 24.
Knee Raises With Barbells at the Sides

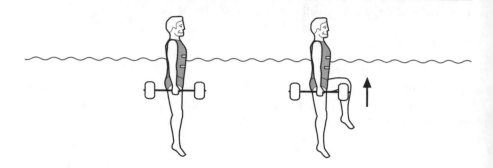

PURPOSE

This exercise improves balance and stimulates and strengthens the arm, thigh, and leg muscles.

EQUIPMENT

Large barbells, flotation vest.

STARTING POSITION

Float vertically with your arms straight down at your sides, holding barbells. Maintain your balance.

ACTION

1. Lift your left knee up high.

2. Bring your leg back down.

3. Lift your right knee up high.

4. Bring your leg back down.

MINDSET

Visualize your knee rising up. Strain to move your leg, and picture the signals passing down through your nerves to the muscles. Feel it tingle.

COMMENTS

Concentrate on maintaining balance as you raise and lower your knee.

Water Exercise 25.
Roll-Overs

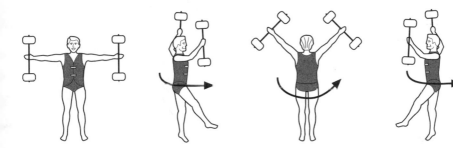

PURPOSE

This exercise stimulates and strengthens the upper and lower body and helps perfect coordination and balance.

EQUIPMENT

Large barbells, flotation vest.

STARTING POSITION

Lie on your back with your arms extended out to the sides with barbells in each hand.

ACTION

1. Roll over on your left side, turning your head and twisting your body to the left. Lift your right arm out of the water and swing it across your chest, creating momentum to help you roll over.

2. Lie face down in the water.

3. Continue rolling over, turning your head and twisting your body to the left. Lift your left arm out of the water and swing it behind you.

4. Return to the starting position.

COMMENTS

Roll to the left, then roll to the right. This exercise should be a vigorous movement through the water. Splash and have fun!

Water Exercise 26.
Straddling the Barbell

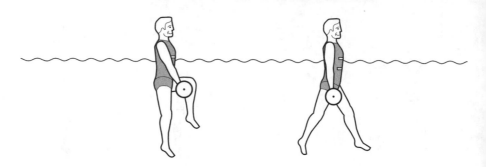

PURPOSE

This exercise improves balance and coordination.

EQUIPMENT

Large barbell, flotation vest.

STARTING POSITION

Float vertically. Place the large barbell under your bent left leg. Put your hands on the Styrofoam floats of the barbell.

ACTION

1. Push the barbell straight down, fully extending your arms. Maintain your balance.

2. Return to the starting position.

3. Repeat this action with the barbell under the other leg.

MINDSET

Imagine that you are a gymnast on a horse.

COMMENTS

At first it will be difficult to balance for any length of time. This exercise requires a lot of upper-body control. To help balance, fix your eyes on a stationary object in the distance, such as a clock on the wall or a tree. Work up to balancing for 25 to 30 seconds at a time.

Water Exercise 27.
Swim and Step

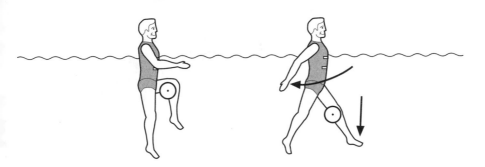

PURPOSE

This exercise improves balance and stimulates leg function.

EQUIPMENT

Large barbell, flotation vest.

STARTING POSITION

Float vertically. Place a large barbell under your bent left knee.

ACTION

1. Use a motion similar to a breaststroke, putting both arms in front of you, cupping your hands, and sweeping your arms behind you in the water.
2. As your arms are moving, push down on the barbell with your left leg, taking a step forward.
3. Let your knee float back up, and return to the starting position.
4. Perform the same action with the barbell under your right knee.

MINDSET

Imagine your leg being able to push the barbell down. Visualize yourself taking a big step.

COMMENTS

Concentrate on pushing your leg down as you step and keeping your upper body in the vertical position.

Water Exercise 28.
Jog in Place With Small Barbells

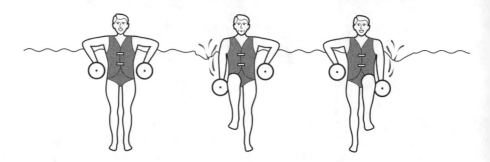

PURPOSE

This exercise stimulates the legs, exercises the arms, and improves coordination.

EQUIPMENT

Small barbells, flotation vest.

STARTING POSITION

Float vertically, holding a small barbell in each hand.

ACTION

Jog in place—bring your left arm up and your right leg down, and vice versa. Coordinate your arm and leg movements.

MINDSET

Visualize that you are jogging in place. As you strain to move your legs, concentrate on coordinating the opposite movements of your arms and legs. Picture the signals passing down through your nerves to the muscles. Feel it tingle.

COMMENTS

Don't swing your arms. Push the barbells straight up and down in the water. Splash and have fun.

Water Exercise 29.
Side Swings With Small Barbells

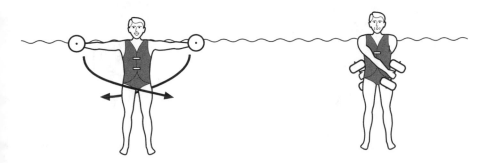

PURPOSE

This exercise improves balance and strengthens the arms.

EQUIPMENT

Small barbells, flotation vest.

STARTING POSITION

Float vertically with your arms extended out to the sides and a bar-bell in each hand.

ACTION

1. Vigorously bring one arm straight down in front and the other arm straight down behind your back. Twist your hands so the barbells are turned to a vertical position in the water.

2. Return your arms to the starting position.

COMMENTS

Perform this exercise over and over again rapidly. Have fun. Splash the water. Maintain body awareness; keep your balance upright.

Water Exercise 30.
Stretch-Outs With Small Barbells

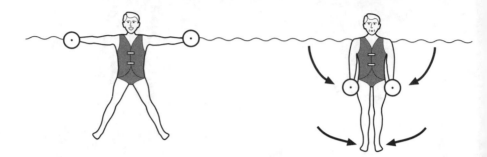

PURPOSE

This exercise improves balance and coordination, strengthens the arms, and stimulates the legs.

EQUIPMENT

Small barbells, flotation vest.

STARTING POSITION

Float vertically with your arms extended out to the sides, holding a small barbell in each hand.

ACTION

1. Stretch your arms and legs out to the sides. Inhale.
2. Swing your arms down to your sides, and bring your legs together. Exhale.

MINDSET

Visualize your legs moving in coordination with your arms. Picture them spreading out wide and coming in together. Think about how each muscle works to make the movements.

COMMENTS

Hold your chin straight. Do this exercise slowly at first, maintaining your balance. Pay attention to breathing deeply. Perform this exercise at different speeds: slow, moderate, and fast.

Water Exercise 31.
Arm Swings With Small Barbells

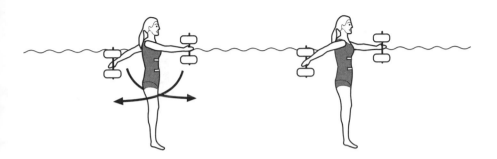

PURPOSE

This exercise improves balance, flexes the shoulders, and strengthens the arms.

EQUIPMENT

Small barbells, flotation vest.

STARTING POSITION

Float vertically. Extend one arm out in front of you and the other arm behind you, holding a small barbell vertically in each hand.

ACTION

1. Swing your arms down and in opposite directions as if walking.

2. Move your arms back and forth.

COMMENTS

Perform this exercise vigorously, splashing. Increase ROM gradually.

Water Exercise 32.
Leg Kicks With Small Barbells

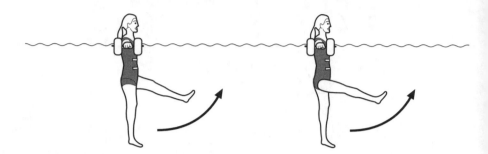

PURPOSE

This exercise stimulates the abdominal, back, and leg muscles.

EQUIPMENT

Small barbells, flotation vest.

STARTING POSITION

Float vertically, holding small barbells straight out to the sides.

ACTION

1. Kick your left leg out in front of you.

2. Return the leg to the starting position.

3. Kick your right leg out in front of you.

4. Return the leg to the starting position.

MINDSET

Imagine that you are playing soccer, kicking a ball high in the air. Visualize your leg coming all the way up. Strain the muscles, and feel your nerves tingle.

COMMENTS

Try to lift your knee and kick out hard with your foot.

Water Exercise 33.
Small Barbell Pass

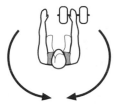 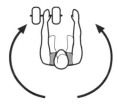

PURPOSE

This exercise increases ROM in the neck, arms, and shoulders and improves balance and coordination.

EQUIPMENT

Small barbell, flotation vest.

STARTING POSITION

Float vertically with your arms stretched out in front of you, holding a small barbell in your right hand.

ACTION

1. Swing both arms out to the sides and reach behind your back. Turn your head to the right. Pass the barbell to your left hand.

2. Swing both arms to the front, turning your head forward. Pass the barbell to your right hand.

COMMENTS

Perform this exercise vigorously. Have fun and splash. Change passing the barbell from left to right and right to left. Alternate the position of your head, turning left and right.

Water Exercise 34.
Barbell Boxing

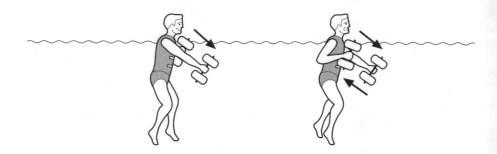

PURPOSE

This exercise improves coordination and flexibility and strengthens your arm and shoulder muscles.

EQUIPMENT

Small barbells, flotation vest.

STARTING POSITION

Float vertically, leaning slightly forward. Hold small barbells in front of you, with your elbows bent.

ACTION

1. Punch your right arm down at an angle into the water.

2. Return your right arm to the starting position, and at the same time punch your left arm down.

3. Alternate arm movements, punching out with one arm and in with the other.

COMMENTS

Exercise vigorously. Have fun and splash. In the beginning, punch down at a slight angle into the water. Increase the difficulty by decreasing the angle to 45 degrees. Vary the exercise by punching out to the sides and in different directions.

Water Exercise 35.
Walking

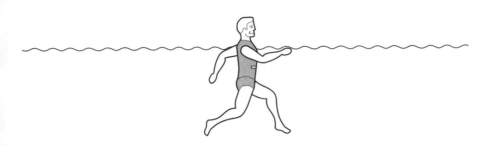

PURPOSE

This exercise strengthens the arms; stimulates the legs; and improves upper-body balance, coordination, and endurance.

EQUIPMENT

Flotation vest.

STARTING POSITION

Float vertically.

ACTION

1. With your body erect, move through the water as if walking. Coordinate your arm and leg movements. As your left arm goes forward, step out with the right foot.

2. As your right arm goes forward, step out with your left foot.

MINDSET

Imagine you are walking. As your arms swing back and forth, visualize your legs moving. Coordinate the movements in your mind. Try to wake up the muscles. Concentrate on making your legs move.

COMMENTS

Pay special attention to remaining vertical in the water. Keep your chin straight. Breathe deeply. Do not cup your hands or use them as paddles. Let your arms and legs do the work. Concentrate on lifting your knees up as you walk.

Start off with short sessions in deep water, where your feet will not touch bottom. As your arms swing, you will move through the water. In the beginning, move forward only a few meters. As your strength and endurance builds, increase the distance you travel. Walk at different speeds: slow, moderate, and fast. A fast walk will give you a real aerobic workout.

Gradually move into chest-deep water, where your feet just touch bottom. Concentrate on pushing your legs down to touch the bottom as you walk. Eventually, move all the way into shallow water and actually walk on your legs.

This is a crucial exercise for those desiring to walk. It is one of the most effective for stimulating your nerves to regenerate. It should be included in almost every workout.

I found it extremely difficult to coordinate the opposite movements of my arms and legs (especially when I could not detect any leg movement). Prior to my accident, I walked without thinking. Now when I try to walk, I have to concentrate on coordinating the movements. This is a mental challenge, as much as a physical one.

Don't be discouraged. Eventually, you will see micro movements in your legs. This is your first step in regaining the ability to walk.

VARIATION

Walk backwards. Exercise in both directions.

Water Exercise 36.
Upright Breaststroke

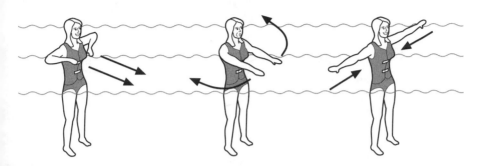

PURPOSE

This exercise strengthens the upper body and increases lung capacity and breathing power.

EQUIPMENT

Flotation vest.

STARTING POSITION

Float vertically.

ACTION

1. Extend your arms straight out in front of you. Inhale.

2. Swing your arms out to the sides, cupping your hands to pull you through the water. Exhale.

3. Bend your arms at the elbows, bringing your hands in close together at the chest.

COMMENTS

Your body will bend forward as you move through the water. This is good. Do not attempt to stay completely vertical. As you build up strength, concentrate on doing the frog kick with your legs, as if swimming the breaststroke. Perform this exercise in both directions— swim backwards.

Water Exercise 37.
Side Stroke

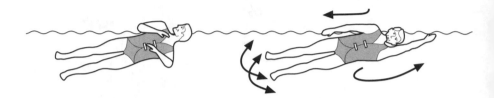

PURPOSE

This exercise will help you strengthen your neck, arm, and upper-body muscles and stimulate the leg muscles.

EQUIPMENT

Flotation vest.

STARTING POSITION

Lie on your left side with your arms bent and your hands by your chest. Inhale.

ACTION

1. Push your left arm out straight, gliding it along the surface. At the same time, cup your right hand and push back, which will move your body forward. Exhale.

2. Cup your left hand and pull it back to your chest, moving your body forward. At the same time, let your right hand glide back up to your chest. Inhale.

3. After swimming some distance on your left side, alternate and do this stroke on your right side.

MINDSET

Visualize your legs moving back and forth, doing the scissor kick. Think about sending the signal down from your brain through your nerves. Visualize the electrical signal stimulating your leg muscles and making them move.

COMMENTS

At first, focus on maintaining your balance on your side and coordinating your arm movements. As you build up strength, concentrate on doing the scissor kick, sweeping your legs back and forth. Try to extend the legs fully horizontally.

Water Exercise 38.
Balancing on Your Side

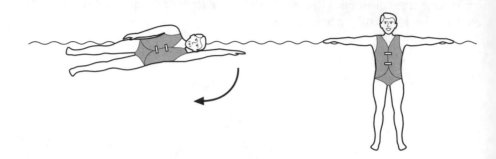

PURPOSE

This exercise strengthens the upper body and improves balance.

EQUIPMENT

Flotation vest.

STARTING POSITION

Lie on your left side with your left arm extended past your head and your right arm against your side.

ACTION

1. Maintain your balance lying on your side for 3 to 5 seconds.

2. Push down forcefully with your left arm and lean up into the vertical position. Let your arms relax and float comfortably in the water.

3. Perform the same exercise on your right side.

COMMENTS

Attempt this exercise after you have mastered the "Side Stretch" exercise (see page 163), which is similar to this exercise, except it uses barbells. Slowly increase the time you stay balanced. At first, it may be difficult to return to the vertical position. When you have mastered this exercise, you should be able to go upright quickly using your arms, legs, and body.

Water Exercise 39.
Pushups in the Corner

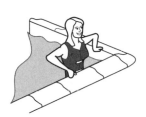 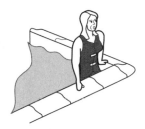

PURPOSE

This exercise strengthens the arms and upper body, improves balance, and stimulates the legs.

EQUIPMENT

Flotation vest.

STARTING POSITION

Stand facing the corner of the pool. Bend your arms at the elbows, holding onto each side.

ACTION

1. Push yourself up out of the pool. Extend your legs down straight.

2. Hold this position for 3 to 5 seconds and return to the starting position.

3. Perform several repetitions. Then turn around, with your back facing the corner, and do pushups.

COMMENTS

Determine how many pushups you can do. Then take two-thirds of that amount and do that number of pushups two or three times. For instance, if you can do twelve pushups, do two or three sets of eight. Increase the number of repetitions as you build up strength. Remove the flotation vest for more of a challenge. As you push up with your arms, push your legs down straight.

Water Exercise 40.
Leg Lifts From the Corner

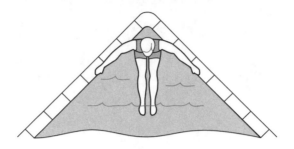

PURPOSE

This exercise stimulates and strengthens the leg, abdominal, and side muscles.

EQUIPMENT

Flotation vest.

STARTING POSITION

Stand with your back in the corner. Extend your arms out along the top edges of the pool.

ACTION

1. Try to swing your legs up together, bending at the hips.

2. Hold this position for 3 to 5 seconds, then lower them back down.

MINDSET

Visualize your legs stretching out straight. Imagine the muscles in your lower back and abdomen working together to help lift the legs and lower them.

COMMENTS

This exercise should be performed regularly early on, even when no movement is detected. Always picture your legs moving in your mind. At first, you will only feel the strain on your arms and upper back. As time progresses, you will feel the strain lower in your back and eventually in your legs.

Water Exercise 41.
Backward Leg Lifts in the Corner

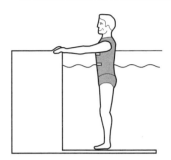 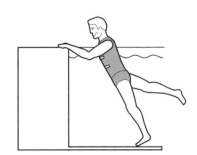

PURPOSE

This exercise stimulates and strengthens the legs.

EQUIPMENT

Flotation vest.

STARTING POSITION

Stand in the shallow end of the pool facing the corner with your arms out straight holding onto each side of the pool. Stand erect with your feet touching the bottom.

ACTION

1. Lean forward and stretch your right leg straight out behind you. Keep your left foot touching the bottom. Hold this position for 5 or 6 seconds.

2. Return to the starting position.

3. Perform the same exercise with your left leg.

MINDSET

Imagine that you are standing on your feet. As you lean forward and raise one leg, see it happening in your mind. Concentrate on sending the signals down from your brain through the nerves and out to the leg muscles.

Water Exercise 42.
Knee Raises at the Wall

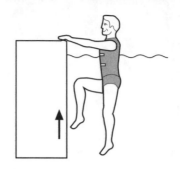

PURPOSE

This exercise stimulates and strengthens the thighs and legs.

EQUIPMENT

Flotation vest.

STARTING POSITION

Stand in deep water, holding the wall of the pool with your arms out straight.

ACTION

1. Lift your right knee up high.

2. Bring your leg back down.

3. Lift your left knee up high.

4. Bring your leg back down.

MINDSET

Imagine raising your knee up high. Visualize it happening in your mind, and strain to wake up those old nerves and muscles.

COMMENTS

Keep your chin straight. At first, it will be difficult to detect any movement. Have an assistant look in the water and let you know how you progress.

Water Exercise 43.
Knee Raises in the Corner

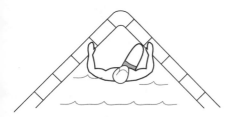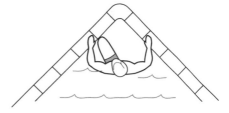

PURPOSE

This exercise stimulates and strengthens the thighs and legs.

EQUIPMENT

Flotation vest.

STARTING POSITION

Hold onto each side of the pool with your body upright.

ACTION

1. Lift your right knee up and touch the wall.

2. Bring your right knee back down.

3. Lift your left knee up and touch the wall.

4. Bring your left knee back down.

MINDSET

As you strain to lift up your knee, visualize your leg rising in the water and touching the wall. Imagine what it feels like when your knee touches the wall. Picture the peripheral nerves in your knee "feeling" the wall and sending the signal back up through the spinal column to the brain.

COMMENTS

Concentrate on each leg. As you raise one, step down with the other.

Water Exercise 44.
Crawling up in the Corner

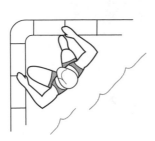 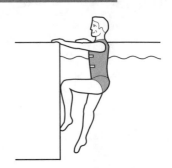

PURPOSE

This exercise stimulates and strengthens the thighs and legs.

EQUIPMENT

Flotation vest.

STARTING POSITION

Stand facing the corner. Bend your arms and hold onto each side of the pool. Let your legs hang loose, with your knees touching the wall.

ACTION

1. Try to climb up the wall. Lift your left leg, bending at the knee, keeping your right leg against the wall.

2. Lift your left leg in the same way and continue climbing up the wall.

3. Keep climbing, alternating legs.

MINDSET

Imagine there is a ladder in the corner. Visualize climbing up, stepping on each rung of the ladder.

COMMENTS

Concentrate on each leg. As you raise one, step down with the other.

Water Exercise 45.
Horizontal Stretch in the Corner

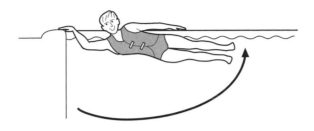

PURPOSE

This exercise stretches the upper body and stimulates and strengthens the legs.

EQUIPMENT

Flotation vest.

STARTING POSITION

Hold your body upright in the deep end of the pool with your back in the corner. Hold onto each side of the pool. Stretch your legs straight down. Your feet should not touch the bottom.

ACTION

1. Swing your legs up against one side of the pool, lying on your side. Stretch your legs out straight and keep them together.

2. Hold this position with your legs up high against the surface.

3. Return to the starting position.

4. Now perform the same action with the opposite side.

Water Exercise 46.
Upright Twist and Turn

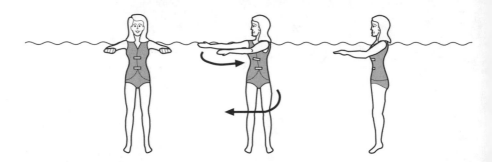

PURPOSE

This exercise strengthens the arms and stretches the sides of the upper body.

EQUIPMENT

Flotation vest.

STARTING POSITION

Hold your body upright in the pool with your arms held out in front of you in a relaxed position.

ACTION

1. Lift your arms just out of the water. Twist your upper body, your head, and your arms to the right.

2. Cup your hands and push down and back in the water as you turn your body 90 degrees to the right. You should now be looking straight ahead with your arms out in front.

3. Repeat this exercise again, turning several times until you end up where you started.

4. Reverse the procedure, this time making turns to the left.

COMMENTS

In the beginning, it will be difficult to turn completely 90 degrees. As you build up strength, it will be easier to turn. Turn vigorously, creating a whirlpool in the water.

Water Exercise 47.
Stand up at the Wall

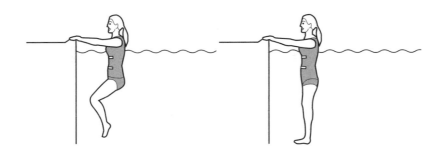

PURPOSE

This exercise stimulates the legs.

EQUIPMENT

Flotation vest.

STARTING POSITION

Choose a depth where your feet will just touch the bottom when your legs are stretched out straight down. Hold onto the edge of the pool with your arms extended, and hold your body upright.

ACTION

1. Try to stand up straight. Stretch your body out and extend your legs down so your feet will touch the bottom.

2. Hold this position for a short while and then relax.

3. Repeat the exercise several times.

COMMENTS

Use your mind to visualize what your legs are doing. Imagine what it feels like to have your feet touch the bottom. Extend your legs, paying attention to your hips, knees, and ankles. Strain hard and feel your nerves tingle.

Water Exercise 48.
Circle Kick

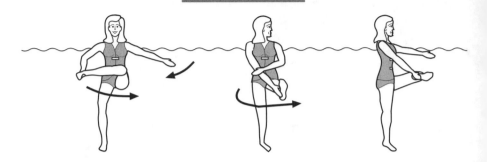

PURPOSE

This exercise stimulates the leg muscles.

EQUIPMENT

Flotation vest.

STARTING POSITION

Hold your body upright. Grab your left foot with your right hand. Hold your foot out in front of your chest. Extend your left arm straight out to the side.

ACTION

1. Turn to the left. While holding your foot, kick your left leg out in the direction of the turn. Help move your leg by pushing your foot to the left with your right hand. Cup your left hand and swing your left arm through the water back in front of you, turning your body to the left.

2. Lift your left arm out of the water, and extend it straight out to your left side, returning to the starting position.

3. Repeat these steps several times until you have made a complete circle to the left.

4. Perform the same exercise in reverse. Hold your right foot in your left hand, and circle to the right.

COMMENTS

Concentrate on kicking your leg out to the side as you turn. Your hand will help push your leg, but watch your leg move and imagine that your leg is actually doing the work.

Water Exercise 49.
Side Step

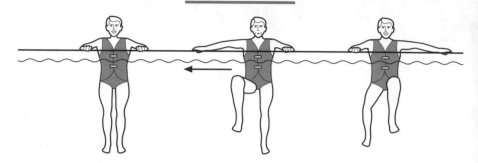

PURPOSE

This exercise stimulates the legs.

EQUIPMENT

Flotation vest.

STARTING POSITION

Hold your body upright in the pool, facing the wall. Hold onto the edge of the pool with both arms out in front of you.

ACTION

1. Lift your right knee up high, and side step out to the right. Reach over with your right arm, grabbing the edge.
2. Lift your left knee high, and side step to the right, bringing your feet together again. As your leg moves, help pull your body along with your right arm.
3. Repeat these steps, moving along the side of the pool.
4. Repeat these actions, moving to the other side.

MINDSET

Imagine that your legs lift up high as you step out and move along.

COMMENTS

At first, most of your movement will be from the arms. Strain your muscles and attempt to lift your knees and move your legs. Use the sides of your upper body to help lift and move the legs.

Water Exercise 50.
Horizontal Stretching at the Ladder

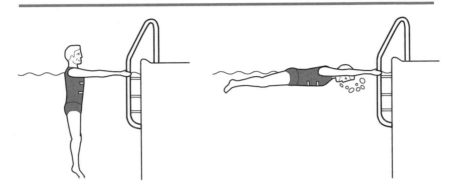

PURPOSE

This exercise works the arms, shoulders, and back and stimulates the legs.

EQUIPMENT

You may wear a flotation vest if you find it necessary, though the vest may make this exercise difficult to do.

STARTING POSITION

Hold your body upright in the pool facing the ladder. Hold onto the ladder with each hand.

ACTION

1. Lie face down in the water. Extend your arms out straight in front of you. Stretch your legs out, and lift them up to the surface.

2. Maintain this position for a short while.

3. Return to the upright position, pulling the legs back down into the water.

COMMENTS

You may find that it is difficult to perform this exercise while wearing a flotation vest. If so, do not wear one, as you will be holding onto a ladder. At first, most of the movement will come from your arms. Concentrate on moving your legs. Over time, you should gradually feel the strain move down from your shoulders and into your back.

Water Exercise 51.
Turning Along the Wall

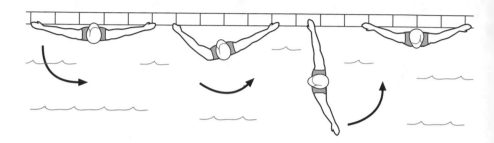

PURPOSE

This exercise works the arms, shoulders, and back and stimulates the upper body.

EQUIPMENT

Flotation vest.

STARTING POSITION

Hold your body upright in the water. Place your chest against the wall. Holding onto the edge of the pool with your arms extended.

ACTION

1. Push off the wall with your left arm.

2. Twist your body around, making a 180-degree turn, so your back is up against the wall.

3. Hold onto the wall with both arms.

4. Swing your right arm out and across your chest.

5. Make another 180-degree turn, so you end up with your chest against the wall.

6. Repeat this exercise several times, advancing along the side of the pool.

7. Do the same in the other direction.

Water Exercise 52.
Catch Your Knee

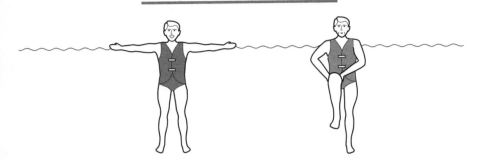

PURPOSE

This exercise stimulates the legs.

EQUIPMENT

Flotation vest.

STARTING POSITION

Hold your body upright in the water. Relax with your arms floating at your sides.

ACTION

1. Raise one knee up high. Swing your arms down into the water, grasp your hands under your thigh, and help raise your leg.

2. Hold your knee up high for a short while.

3. Release your arms and lower your leg back down. Use your hands to help push down on your leg.

4. Repeat this exercise, alternating legs.

COMMENTS

This is an exercise for the mind as much as it is for the legs. Perform this exercise every time you work out in the pool. Picture your leg moving up and down without the assistance of your hands. You are training your mind to make the nerves and muscles work, as you see your leg move through the water.

Water Exercise 53.
Balance With the Kickboard

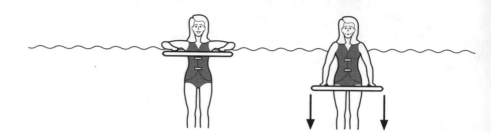

PURPOSE

This exercise improves balance and strengthens the upper arms.

EQUIPMENT

Kickboard, flotation vest.

STARTING POSITION

Hold your body upright in the water. Turn the kickboard sideways in the water in front of your chest. Place both hands on top of the kickboard.

ACTION

1. Push the kickboard down slowly into the water, extending your arms.

2. Hold this position for a short while, maintaining your balance.

3. Bring the kickboard slowly back up to the surface.

Water Exercise 54.
Vertical Kickboard Strokes

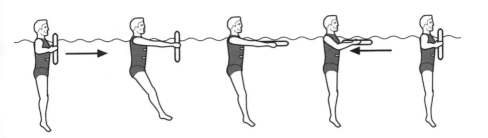

PURPOSE

This exercise strengthens the upper arms.

EQUIPMENT

Kickboard, flotation vest.

STARTING POSITION

Hold your body upright in the water. Grasp onto either end of the kickboard. Hold the kickboard vertically against your chest.

ACTION

1. Push the kickboard out in front on you. This will move you backwards through the water.

2. Turn the kickboard flat on the surface and pull your arms back in.

3. Rotate the kickboard vertically and repeat the exercise.

4. Perform the exercise in reverse and move forward through the water.

Water Exercise 55.
Kickboard Twist

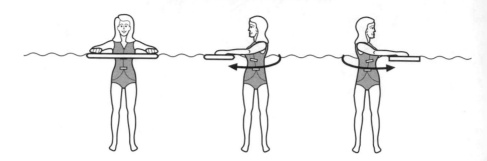

PURPOSE

This exercise improves ROM and stimulates leg movement.

EQUIPMENT

Kickboard, flotation vest.

STARTING POSITION

Float vertically, holding the kickboard flat on the water surface. With your arms out in front of you, place one hand flat on each end of the kickboard.

ACTION

1. Twist your upper body to the left, gliding the kickboard over the surface. Attempt to twist your hips and legs to the right.

2. Twist your upper body to the right, gliding the kickboard over the surface. Attempt to twist your hips and legs to the left.

MINDSET

As you twist your upper body through the water, visualize your legs and hips twisting in the opposite direction. Picture the signals from the brain going down through your nerves to move your legs.

Water Exercise 56.
Push to the Rear

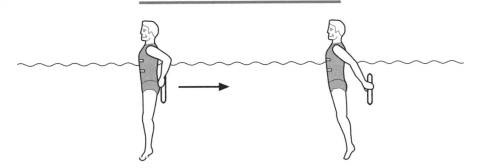

PURPOSE

This exercise improves balance and stability and strengthens the shoulder and abdominal muscles.

EQUIPMENT

Kickboard, flotation vest.

STARTING POSITION

Float vertically. Place your arms behind your back, and hold the kickboard vertically against your buttocks.

ACTION

1. Push the kickboard back away from you, extending your arms. Hold this position for 2 to 3 seconds.

2. Pull the kickboard in against your buttocks. Hold this position for 2 to 3 seconds.

COMMENTS

As you move the kickboard, maintain your balance and keep your body vertical in the water. To help maintain your balance, focus your eyes on one spot in the distance, such as a clock on the wall. Perform this exercise at different speeds: slow, moderate pace, and fast. At medium and fast speeds, move your arms continuously back and forth without holding your arms in the extended position.

Water Exercise 57.
Prone Pushups

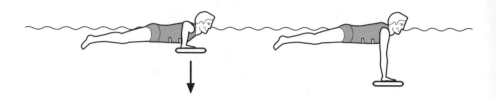

PURPOSE

This exercise strengthens the arm muscles and improves balance and stability.

EQUIPMENT

Kickboard, flotation vest.

STARTING POSITION

Lie on your stomach in the water. Position the kickboard just under your chest with both hands placed flat on it.

ACTION

1. Slowly extend your arms, pushing the kickboard down. Hold it there for 2 to 3 seconds. Exhale as you extend your arms.

2. Slowly retract your arms, bringing the kickboard up against your chest. Inhale as you retract your arms.

COMMENTS

You can grasp the edges of the kickboard with each hand for more control. As your balance and control improve, place your hands flat on top. Do not let the kickboard wobble. Concentrate on keeping it horizontal as you move through the water.

Visualize your back as completely straight with your stomach in. Concentrate on your breathing.

Water Exercise 58.
Backward Breaststroke

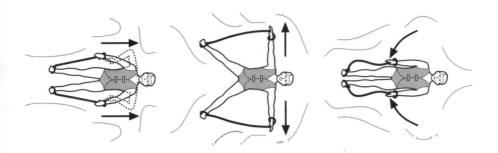

PURPOSE

This exercise strengthens the upper body and stimulates the legs.

EQUIPMENT

Two pieces of tubing of equal length, flotation vest. To determine the length of your tubing, lie on your back with your arms stretched out to the sides and your legs spread apart. The tubing should reach from your right hand to your right foot without any slack.

STARTING POSITION

Lie flat on your back in the pool. Attach the tubing from your hands to your feet. Bring your legs together and keep your arms down at your sides.

ACTION

1. Bring your arms straight out the sides, gliding them over the surface of the water. Spread your legs apart. Inhale.

2. Cup your hands and pull your arms down through the water to your sides. Bring your legs together. Exhale.

3. With these movements, you will be swimming. Start off by swimming a short distance. As your endurance increases, swim several laps.

COMMENTS

In the beginning, your arms will pull your legs apart with the tubing. Picture your legs moving in your mind without the tubing. Concentrate on moving your legs. You are reteaching your body how to work.

Water Exercise 59.
Swim With Short Tubing

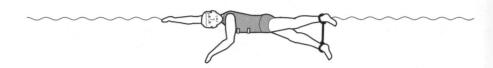

PURPOSE

This exercise strengthens the leg muscles.

EQUIPMENT

Exercise tubing, flotation vest.

STARTING POSITION

Slip your feet through the loops in the end of the exercise tubing, and slide it up around your ankles. Float horizontally.

ACTION

Swim using the "American Crawl" (see page 173). As you kick, try to stretch the tubing.

MINDSET

Visualize your legs kicking in the water. Imagine feeling the exercise tubing and stretching it out as you move your legs.

COMMENTS

At first, you may not have any leg movement. As your control improves, use the resistance of the tubing to exercise your muscles. Perform this exercise using the backstroke and side stroke.

Water Exercise 60.
Swim With Attached Tubing

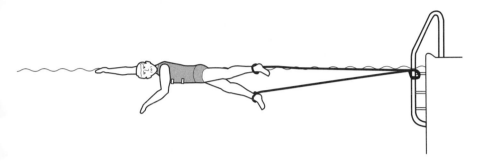

PURPOSE

This exercise strengthens the arm and leg muscles.

EQUIPMENT

Exercise tubing, flotation vest.

STARTING POSITION

Attach one end of the first piece of tubing to a stationary object, like the pool ladder. Attach the other end to your right ankle. Attach the other piece of tubing to a stationary object and your left ankle. Float vertically in deep water.

ACTION

Swim using the "American Crawl" (see page 173). Try to swim away from the stationary object, stretching the tubing.

MINDSET

Visualize your legs kicking in the water. Imagine feeling the exercise tubing and stretching it out as you move your legs. In your mind, coordinate the movement of your arms with the kicking of your legs.

COMMENTS

As you move farther away, the tubing will stretch, providing resistance. You should eventually be able to swim in place. Try to swim away from the object for 30 seconds to one minute.

Conclusion

W hile millions of dollars are being spent in traditional medical research to find a possible cure for paralysis through nerve transplants or other invasive surgical techniques, many people are taking a natural approach to healing themselves. It is amazing to us that the medical community has not recognized that many people have cured themselves through sheer determination, willpower, proper diet, and exercise.

For over forty years, Dr. Burdenko has been developing his unique method of physical training, conditioning, and rehabilitation into a program he calls the Burdenko Method. Although this was not originally intended to treat paralysis, Dr. Burdenko learned that the same techniques and philosophy he employed to rehabilitate professional and amateur athletes recovering from injury provided surprising and remarkable results for paralyzed patients. As I started working with Dr. Burdenko, we began documenting his techniques so that he would have something to give to other patients like me. The result has been this book, which documents my experience learning his philosophy and performing his exercises—learning how to help my body through the natural healing process. I am following in the footsteps of others who were paralyzed even more severely than myself, who now walk freely on their own.

I am still following my rehabilitation program. Exercising in the pool recently, I actually saw my legs move again as I strained to bring life back into my limbs. It is only a matter of time before I will have full function of my body.

If you are paralyzed and you truly desire to walk again, the main thing that stands in your way is the courage to go ahead with this program. It takes a lot of hard work and dedication, but it can be done. The results of this program may vary. Some will be able to completely walk away from their wheelchairs. Others will be able to improve their health and their level of conditioning. The degree to which you can succeed is up to you. So get out there and do it!

I wish you the best of luck in pursuing your goals. Thank you for letting us share our experience with the Burdenko Method. This is the best way I know of to give you the opportunity to get involved in a program that may change your life forever. Never give up!

Suggested Readings

Anderson, R.A. and D.G. Bornell. *Stretch & Strengthen*. Palmer Lake, CO: Shelter Publications, 1984.

Bates, A. and N. Hanson. *Aquatic Exercise Therapy*. Canada: Online Graphics, 1992.

Brooks, G. A. and T.D. Fahey. *Exercise Physiology: Human Bioenergetics and Its Applications*. New York: John Wiley & Sons, 1984.

Burdenko, I.N. and E.A. Connors. *The Ultimate Power of Resistance*. Boston: Igor Inc., 1991.

Carlson, R. *Don't Sweat the Small Stuff*. New York: Hyperion, 1997.

Cratty, B. *Adapted Physical Education for Handicapped Children and Youth*. Denver: Love Publishing Co., 1980.

Feldenkrais, M. *Awareness Through Movement*. New York: Harper and Row, 1977.

Huey, L. and R. Forster. *The Complete Waterpower Workout Book*. New York: Random House, 1993.

Krasevec, J.A. and D.C. Grimes. *HydroRobics*. West Point, NY: Leisure Press, 1985.

Maddox, S. *Spinal Network: The Total Resource for the Wheelchair Community*, Malibu, CA: Miramar Communications, 1990.

McArdle, W.D., F.I. Katch, and V.L. Katch. *Exercise Physiology: Energy, Nutrition, and Human Performance*. London: Lea & Febiger, 1981.

McWaters, J.G. *Deep-Water Exercise for Health and Fitness.* Laguna Beach, CA: Publitec Editions, 1988.

Smith, P. *Total Breathing.* New York: McGraw Hill Paperbacks, 1980.

Southmayd, W. and M. Hoffman. *Sports Health: The Complete Book of Athletic Injuries.* New York: The Putnam Publishing Group, 1981.

Stoler, D.R. and B. Albers Hill. *Coping With Mild Traumatic Brain Injury.* Garden City Park, NY: Avery Publishing Group, 1998.

Watkins, R.G., B. Buhler, and P. Loverlock. *The Water Workout Recovery Program.* Chicago: Contemporary Books, 1988.

Weil, A. *Spontaneous Healing: How to Discover and Enhance Your Body's Natural Ability to Heal Itself.* New York: Ballantine Books, 1996.

About the Authors

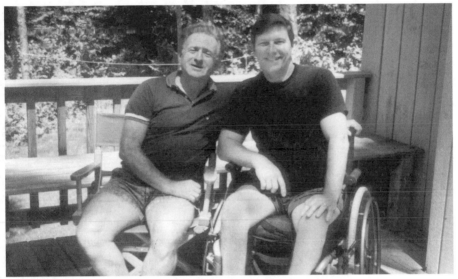

Dr. Igor Burdenko and Scott Biehler

Dr. Igor Burdenko received his doctorate in Sports Medicine in his native Russia, where he was an athlete, trainer, coach, and sports medicine professional. He is a member of the American College of Sports Medicine. Today, he runs the Water and Sports Therapy Institute in Boston, Massachusetts. Dr. Burdenko has received numerous awards for his work and has a long list of prestigious clients, including Olympic silver-medalist Nancy Kerrigan, former Boston Celtic Kevin McHale, and Olympic gold-medalist Oksana Baiul.

Scott Biehler received his bachelor's degree from Auburn University in Auburn Alabama. Prior to his accident, he was an account manager for a computer graphics software company in Boston. He currently lives in a suburb of central Florida, where he is still following the Burdenko Method and improving day by day.

Index

Healthy Habits

are easy to come by—

IF YOU KNOW WHERE TO LOOK!

Get the latest information on:

- **better health • diet & weight loss**
- **the latest nutritional supplements**
- **herbal healing • homeopathy and more**

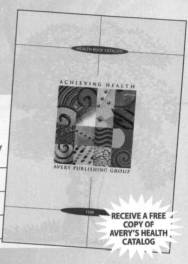

COMPLETE AND RETURN THIS CARD RIGHT AWAY!

Where did you purchase this book?

- ❏ bookstore
- ❏ health food store
- ❏ pharmacy
- ❏ supermarket
- ❏ other (please specify)_____

Name_____

Street Address_____

City_____ State_____ Zip_____

RECEIVE A FREE COPY OF AVERY'S HEALTH CATALOG

GIVE ONE TO A FRIEND ...

Healthy Habits

are easy to come by—

IF YOU KNOW WHERE TO LOOK!

Get the latest information on:

- **better health • diet & weight loss**
- **the latest nutritional supplements**
- **herbal healing • homeopathy and more**

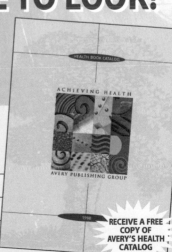

COMPLETE AND RETURN THIS CARD RIGHT AWAY!

Where did you purchase this book?

- ❏ bookstore
- ❏ health food store
- ❏ pharmacy
- ❏ supermarket
- ❏ other (please specify)_____

Name_____

Street Address_____

City_____ State_____ Zip_____

RECEIVE A FREE COPY OF AVERY'S HEALTH CATALOG

Avery Publishing Group

120 Old Broadway
Garden City Park, NY 11040

Avery Publishing Group

120 Old Broadway
Garden City Park, NY 11040